FOURTH EDITION

MAYO CLINIC

Diet Manual

BY THE COMMITTEE
ON DIETETICS
OF
THE MAYO CLINIC

W. B. Saunders Company
PHILADELPHIA • LONDON • TORONTO

W. B. Saunders Company: West Washington Square
Philadelphia, Pa. 19105

12 Dyott Street
London, WC1A 1DB

833 Oxford Street
Toronto 18, Ontario

Mayo Clinic Diet Manual   ISBN 0-7216-6211-0

Print No.:   9   8   7   6   5   4

PREFACE
TO THE FOURTH EDITION

The dietary procedures outlined in this book were developed for the guidance of staff, resident and intern physicians, dietitians, dietetic interns and nurses of the Mayo Foundation, the Mayo Clinic, and the associated hospitals of this clinic in Rochester, Minnesota. They are described in technical terms and are designed for use by persons with training in medicine or dietetics. They are not intended for direct distribution to patients.

The diets represent the convergent trend, but not unanimity, of opinion of the physicians of the Clinic. When prescribing diets, physicians of the Clinic are requested to base their orders on the standard diets as outlined, individualizing them by ordering the appropriate standard diet or combination of standard diets with such modification as they consider necessary to meet the particular needs of the individual patient. It should be emphasized that the diets as outlined should serve only as a guide to physicians ordering diets and to dietitians planning and serving food for patients. It is obviously essential that the food served be eaten if the diet is to be of value to the patient. For this reason, it is important to make sure not only that the proper types and amounts of foods are served but also that the foods are served in such a way that the patient will eat them.

Tables of approximate composition of foods published in the U. S. Department of Agriculture Handbook No. 8* were used in planning these diets, except as indicated in the text.

Since the appearance of the third edition of the *Mayo Clinic Diet Manual* (1961), many changes have occurred as a result of new knowledge of diseases and advances in the science of nutrition. However, in keeping with the acknowledgment that numerous phases of diet therapy are still based on traditional practice rather than on scientific fact, a general effort has been made toward liberalization wherever it seemed indicated. Because of increased emphasis on reduction of cholesterol and saturated fats in the American diet, the general and therapeutic diets in the manual are planned so that fat contributes 40% or less of the calories, with stress being placed on fewer foods containing saturated fats and cholesterol. A section devoted to diets controlled in protein, sodium, and potassium for the management of renal disease has been added. Diets for the pediatric

---

*U. S. Department of Agriculture. Composition of Foods—Raw, Processed, Prepared. U. S. Department of Agriculture Handbook No. 8, revised December 1963.

age group now appear as a separate section. The diet for disorders of the gallbladder has been deleted, as have the dietary regimens for anorexia nervosa. The gluten-restricted diet for sprue has been liberalized in its fat and residue content. Our dietary program for ulcerative colitis places less emphasis on intermediate stages. Diets for peptic ulcer have been simplified by deletion of some of the stricter programs, and they have been liberalized generally as well as reduced in fat content. New diets for use during pregnancy have been devised. The diets for management of gout also have been rewritten. A fundamental change in the present edition is the use of the Mayo Clinic Food Exchange List, which is derived from the American Diabetes Association Food Exchange List, as the basis for the planning of all therapeutic diets with the exception of the ketogenic and the renal diets. Many minor changes have been made throughout the text as well as in the format.

Diet plans variously called "Mayo Diet," "Mayo Clinic Two-Week Diet," or "Mayo Clinic Egg Diet" have been circulated widely throughout the United States. **These diets did not originate at the Mayo Clinic and have never been used or sanctioned by the Clinic or any of its associated hospitals.** The dietary programs for obesity prescribed and used at this clinic are outlined on pages 71 through 73.

The collaborative effort and consistent counsel of all dietitians of the Mayo Clinic, associated hospitals, and Rochester Diet Kitchen have made this edition possible. Sister Mary Victor, Miss Florence C. Schmidt, and Mrs. Beverly Devney represented St. Marys Hospital; Miss Leota Davis and Mrs. Collette Heise, the Rochester Diet Kitchen and the Rochester Methodist Hospital; Miss Juliette Vernet and Miss Patricia Hodgson, the Mayo Clinic. Mrs. Joyce Margie prepared the portion of the manual on dietary programs for renal disease, which is a major contribution of scientific merit. Miss Hodgson has borne the major load in the work of revision. We are indebted to Mrs. Barbara Peters for typing the copies of the diets that were circulated to the physicians, dietitians, and committee members for their approval. Miss Florence L. Schmidt, Editor in the Section of Publications of the Mayo Clinic, has been of great assistance in the preparation of the manuscript for publication.

Every effort has been made to make this new revision as complete and as accurate as possible and to make it representative of the current dietary practices at the Mayo Clinic and the associated hospitals.

MAYO CLINIC COMMITTEE ON DIETETICS

CONTENTS

SECTION 4   STANDARD HOSPITAL DIETS FOR CHILDREN

APPENDIX

SECTION 1

GENERAL INFORMATION

NUTRITIONAL ADEQUACY OF DIETS

The Recommended Daily Dietary Allowances (1968) of the National Research Council served as a guideline in assessment of the nutritional adequacy of the diets. A Food Composition Table (page 132), which was developed with the use of a computer, was used in analyzing the diets. The following policy was established in describing the nutritional adequacy of each diet:

1. The nutritive composition of each diet was compared to the mean nutrient requirements for the average Mayo Clinic patient who is a patient 50 years of age. The figures used for average height and weight correspond to those for males and females listed in the Recommended Daily Dietary Allowances (page 130) of the National Research Council.

2. A statement of nutritional adequacy was not included in the discussion of the diet if it met the recommended allowances for the average Mayo Clinic patient.

3. A statement of nutritional adequacy was included if the diet did not meet the recommended allowances for a specific nutrient or nutrients.

As proposed by the National Research Council, the Recommended Daily Dietary Allowances should be used only as a guide in planning nutritionally adequate diets. The Council suggests that a diet should not be considered inadequate if it does not meet the recommended levels. Except for calories, the allowances were designed "to afford a margin sufficiently above average physiological requirements to cover variations among practically all individuals in the general population."

The meal plans included with each diet may be inadequate in iron for women less than 55 years of age. Women for whom such a diet is prescribed should be encouraged to eat foods rich in iron. The physician may wish to prescribe iron supplementation in addition to the foregoing recommended foods.

FORMAT OF DIETS

The format of each diet presented in the manual is similar. In addition to the policies stated under "Nutritional Adequacy of Diets," the following guidelines are used:

1. An initial statement concerning "Nutritional Adequacy" is made only when a diet is low or inadequate in a specific nutrient or nutrients. With certain diets used in the treatment of malabsorption, a statement is made indicating that a physician may wish to order vitamin and mineral supplementation even though the diet is nutritionally adequate.

2. The "Approximate Composition" of the diet is given in a table listing values for protein, fat, carbohydrate, calories, sodium, potassium, and fluid. A variation of 10 to 15% is assumed for the listed values.

3. "General Information" is presented concerning the diet or diets included in the dietary regimen.

4. A table on "Suggested Daily Food Exchanges" is included for each dietary program. Food allowances are specified according to the Mayo Clinic Food Exchange List (front and back end sheets*). Each table on daily food exchanges is to be used only as a guide in planning specific diets. The professional person using the table should make appropriate modifications within the prescribed dietary program in order to adapt the diet to the usual menu patterns of the hospital or to the individual needs of the patient.

5. A "Suggested Menu Pattern" is included for most diets within a dietary program with **approximate amounts** of foods in each instance. Exceptions are made in certain diets in which one pattern is deemed acceptable.

6. In the discussion of foods to be allowed or to be omitted, the foods are grouped as outlined in the Mayo Clinic Food Exchange List. Within each particular food group, minimal words are used in giving the dietary prescription. Headings for food groups are repeated only when necessary for comprehension.

*Throughout the rest of the manual the reference is given as "inside covers."

PLANNING OF GENERAL AND THERAPEUTIC DIETS

A DAILY FOOD GUIDE

The daily diet pattern for general, therapeutic, and home dismissal diets is planned with the Basic Four Food Groups (milk, meat, vegetable-fruit, and bread-cereal) as a guide.

Milk Group   Children and adolescents, 3–4 cups
                                                 Adults, 2 cups

Meat Group   2 servings
Meat, fish, fowl, eggs, cheese, peanut butter

Vegetable-Fruit Group   4 servings
One serving each day:
   Vegetable: a dark green or a yellow
     vegetable for vitamin A
   Fruit: Citrus or other fruit rich in vitamin C

Bread-Cereal Group   4 or more servings
Bread, cereal, potato, potato substitutes

For adults, diets without calorie modifications are planned with approximately 2,055 calories. The energy requirements for older men and women are averaged to obtain the calorie level of 2,055. This level of calories reflects the reduction in calorie allowances associated with advancing age proposed by the National Research Council.

Fats, desserts, and additional servings of basic foods supplement the diet. The diets are planned with 40% or less of the total calories from fat.

SECTION 2

STANDARD HOSPITAL DIETS

GENERAL, SOFT, CLEAR LIQUID, AND FULL LIQUID DIETS

GENERAL DIET

APPROXIMATE COMPOSITION (10 to 15% Variation)

Protein	Fat	Carbohydrate	Calories	Sodium*	Potassium	Fluid
gm	gm	gm		mEq	mEq	ml
70	95	230	2,055	110	80	2,000

*Value is for average amount of salt used in preparation of food; salt added to food at the table is not calculated.

GENERAL INFORMATION

The General Diet may be ordered for the adult patient for whom dietary modifications are not necessary. It includes a wide variety of foods. The diet is planned with approximately 40% of the calories from fat.

The General Diet is planned with the use of the Mayo Clinic Food Exchange List. Servings of food exchanges which would provide a nutritionally adequate diet for adults are suggested in the table that follows. This table should be used only as a guide in planning the diet. Modifications may be made in order to adapt the diet to the normal dietary pattern of the hospital or to the needs of the patient.

SUGGESTED DAILY FOOD EXCHANGES* (Mayo Clinic Food Exchange List, inside covers)

Meat	Fat	Milk	Bread	Vegetable	Fruit	Dessert	Sweets
5	9	2	6	3–4	2–3	1	4

*Amount not restricted.

SUGGESTED MENU PATTERN

Breakfast		Noon Meal		Evening Meal	
Fruit	1 serving	Meat	2 ounces	Meat	2 ounces
Egg	1	Potato	1 serving	Potato	1 serving
Cereal	1 serving	Vegetable	1 serving	Vegetable	1 serving
Toast	1 slice	Salad	1 serving	Salad	1 serving
Fat	3 teaspoons	Bread	1 slice	Bread	1 slice
Sugar, jelly	2 tablespoons	Fat	3 teaspoons	Fat	3 teaspoons
Beverage	1 cup	Fruit	1 serving	Dessert	1 serving
		Milk	1 cup	Milk	1 cup
		Sugar, jelly	1 tablespoon	Sugar, jelly	1 tablespoon
		Beverage	1 cup	Beverage	1 cup

SOFT DIET

APPROXIMATE COMPOSITION (10 to 15% Variation)

Protein	Fat	Carbohydrate	Calories	Sodium*	Potassium	Fluid
gm	gm	gm		mEq	mEq	ml
70	95	230	2,055	110	75	2,000

*Value is for average amount of salt used in preparation of food; salt added to food at the table is not calculated.

GENERAL INFORMATION

The Soft Diet is similar to the General Diet except that foods with indigestible carbohydrates are restricted and meats or shellfish with tough connective tissue are omitted. The diet may be ordered as a progression step from the Full Liquid Diet to the General Diet or as a postoperative diet until the General Diet can be tolerated.

A mechanically soft diet may be ordered for a patient who has difficulty in chewing. Foods modified in texture, such as ground meats and puréed fruits and vegetables, are served.

The Soft Diet is planned with the Mayo Clinic Food Exchange List. Servings of food exchanges are suggested in the following table. This table should be used only as a guide in planning the diets. Modifications within the prescribed dietary restrictions may be made in order to adapt the diet to the normal dietary pattern of the hospital or to the needs of the patient.

SUGGESTED DAILY FOOD EXCHANGES* (Mayo Clinic Food Exchange List, inside covers)

Meat	Fat	Milk	Bread	Vegetable	Fruit	Dessert	Sweets
5	9	2	6	2 (purée or juice)	2–3	1	4

*Amount not restricted.

SUGGESTED MENU PATTERN

Breakfast		Noon Meal		Evening Meal	
Fruit	1 serving	Meat	2 ounces	Meat	2 ounces
Egg	1	Potato	1 serving	Potato	1 serving
Cereal	1 serving	Vegetable*	1 serving	Vegetable*	1 serving
Toast	1 slice	Bread	1 slice	Bread	1 slice
Fat	3 teaspoons	Fat	3 teaspoons	Fat	3 teaspoons
Sugar, jelly	2 tablespoons	Fruit	1 serving	Dessert	1 serving
Beverage	1 cup	Milk	1 cup	Milk	1 cup
		Sugar, jelly	1 tablespoon	Sugar, jelly	1 tablespoon
		Beverage	1 cup	Beverage	1 cup

*Purée or juice.

FOOD GROUPS

Allowed	Omitted
	Fried and highly seasoned foods
Beverage	
Coffee, tea; carbonated beverage; cereal beverage	
Meat	
Meat, fish, or fowl; eggs; cottage cheese, mild cheese used as flavoring	Fried; meat and shellfish with tough connective tissue; other cheese
Fat	
Any except "Omitted"	Avocado; nuts; olives; salad dressing with "Omitted" seasonings
Milk	
Milk, milk drinks	
Bread	
Refined wheat or rye bread, rolls, or crackers; quick breads	Any with whole grain or graham flour, bran, seeds, or nuts
Refined cereals: cooked or ready to eat	Whole grain or bran cereals
Potato and potato substitutes except "Omitted"; puréed corn, lima beans, peas; hominy grits	Potato chips, fried potatoes, whole grain rice; dried legumes; popcorn
Vegetable	
Mild-flavored vegetables: purée or juice	Any other
Fruit	
Canned or cooked fruit or juice: without seeds or tough skin; banana, citrus fruits without membrane	Any other
Soup	
Broth, bouillon; cream soup with "Allowed" foods	Any other
Dessert	
Any except "Omitted"	Any with coconut, nuts, or "Omitted" fruits; pastries
Sweets	
Any except "Omitted"	Jam, marmalade; candy with coconut, nuts, or "Omitted" fruits
Miscellaneous	
Salt; spices, herbs except "Omitted"; chocolate, cocoa; gravy, white sauce; vinegar	Seed spices, garlic; condiments; pickles

CLEAR LIQUID AND FULL LIQUID DIETS

NUTRITIONAL ADEQUACY

The Clear Liquid Diet is adequate only in ascorbic acid.
The Full Liquid Diet is adequate only in calcium and ascorbic acid.

APPROXIMATE COMPOSITION (10 to 15% Variation)

Diet	Protein gm	Fat gm	Carbohydrate gm	Calories	Sodium* mEq	Potassium mEq	Fluid ml
Clear Liquid	10	. . .	135	600	35	35	2,000
Full Liquid	45	60	240	1,700	95	85	2,500

*Value is for amount of salt used in preparation of food; salt added to food at the table is not calculated.

GENERAL INFORMATION

The Clear Liquid Diet and the Full Liquid Diet should be used for short periods only. If a patient receives a liquid diet for more than a week, the physician may wish to order a vitamin supplement (page 134). Between-meal feedings are given routinely at midmorning, midafternoon, and in the evening.

Clear Liquid Diet.   The diet provides minimal residue as it consists only of clear fluids. It may be ordered when it is necessary to restrict the amount of undigested material in the gastrointestinal tract.

Full Liquid Diet.   The diet includes beverages and other foods which liquefy at body temperature. It may be ordered for a patient who is unable to tolerate solid foods.

SUGGESTED MENU PATTERN

	Clear Liquid Diet*	Full Liquid Diet*
Breakfast		
Fruit juice	1 serving	1 serving
Cereal	. . .	1 serving
Fat	. . .	1/3 cup half and half
Sugar	1–2 teaspoons	2 teaspoons
Beverage	1 cup	1 cup
Noon Meal		
Soup	1 serving (broth)	1 serving
Dessert	1 serving	1 serving
Milk or milk drink	. . .	1 cup
Sugar	1–2 teaspoons	2 teaspoons
Beverage	1 cup	1 cup
Evening Meal		
Soup	1 serving (broth)	1 serving (broth)
Dessert	1 serving	1 serving
Milk or milk drink	. . .	1 cup
Sugar	1–2 teaspoons	2 teaspoons
Beverage	1 cup	1 cup
Between-Meal Feedings		
Midmorning		
Fruit juice	1 cup	1 cup
Midafternoon		
Fruit juice	1 cup	. . .
Milk drink (eggnog)	. . .	1 cup
Evening		
Fruit juice	1 cup	1 cup

*Amounts not restricted.

FOOD GROUPS

Clear Liquid Diet	Full Liquid Diet
Allowed: Only foods listed	*Allowed: Only foods listed*

Beverage
Coffee, tea; carbonated beverage; cereal beverage

Beverage
Coffee, tea; carbonated beverage; cereal beverage

Vegetable
Tomato juice

Egg
Dried egg powder: custard, eggnog

Fruit
Fruit juice, strained

Fat
Butter; margarine; half and half

Soup
Broth, bouillon

Milk
Milk, milk drinks

Dessert
Gelatin; fruit ice

Bread
Cooked cereals

Sweets
Sugar; plain sugar candy

Vegetable
Vegetable juice or puréed, mild-flavored vegetables in soups

Miscellaneous
Salt, spices

Fruit
Fruit juice, strained

Soup
Broth, bouillon; cream soup, strained

Dessert
Custard, gelatin, pudding ice cream, sherbet (without coconut, nuts, or whole fruit)

Sweets
Sugar, plain sugar candy

Miscellaneous
Salt, spices; cocoa, chocolate

SECTION 3

DIETARY PROGRAMS FOR THERAPEUTIC DIETS

CARDIOVASCULAR DISEASES

CHOLESTEROL-CONTROLLED DIETS

APPROXIMATE COMPOSITION (10 to 15% Variation)

Diet	Protein gm	Fat gm	Carbohydrate gm	Calories*	Sodium† mEq	Potassium mEq	Fluid ml
Low Cholesterol	75	75	260	2,000	125	80	2,050
Low Cholesterol, No Free Sugar	90	75	245	2,000	150	108	2,400

* Calorie level should be varied according to the calorie requirements for maintenance of ideal weight of the patient.

† Value is for average amount of salt used in preparation of food; salt which may be added to food at the table is not calculated.

GENERAL INFORMATION

Cholesterol-Controlled Diets are planned with a daily intake of 200 mg or less of cholesterol. Inclusion of egg yolks in the diet is not recommended. A moderate amount of liquid vegetable oils, preferably corn or safflower oil, is necessary to meet the recommended level of polyunsaturated fat. Descriptions of diet with modifications of fat and of simple carbohydrates follow:

Low Cholesterol Diet. The **amount** and **kind** of fat are carefully controlled in this diet. The diets are planned with daily cholesterol intake of 200 mg or less. The percentage of fat in the diet is between 30 and 35% of the total calories, with the intake of saturated fat less than 10%. The ratio of polyunsaturated fat to saturated fat is approximately 1:1.

Low Cholesterol, No Free Sugar. The **amount** and **kind** of fat in this diet are carefully controlled. The diets are planned with a daily cholesterol intake of 200 mg or less. The percentage of fat in the diet is between 30 and 35% of the total calories, with the intake of saturated fat less than 10%. The ratio of polyunsaturated fat to saturated fat is approximately 1:1. Simple carbohydrates are restricted by eliminating sugar from the diet and restricting the intake of foods containing simple sugars.

Control of weight usually is recommended for most patients. Therefore, the calorie level of the diet should be varied according to the patient's ideal weight, age, and sex (pages 152-159).

In planning a weight-maintenance diet, it is important to make appropriate calorie modifications. The ratio of polyunsaturated fat to saturated fat of approximately 1:1 should be maintained. The fat content of the diet should not exceed 35% of the total calories.

These diets are planned with the use of the Mayo Clinic Food Exchange List. Servings of food exchanges are suggested in the following Table. This Table should be used only as a guide in planning the diets. Modifications within the prescribed dietary restrictions may be made in order to adapt the diet to the usual menu pattern of the hospital and to the calorie requirements and normal eating pattern of the patient.

SUGGESTED DAILY FOOD EXCHANGES (Mayo Clinic Food Exchange List, inside covers)

Diet	Meat	Fat	Skim milk	Bread	Vegetable	Fruit	Dessert	Sweets
Low Cholesterol	6*	9†	2‡	7‡	3–4‡	4‡	1‡	3‡
Low Cholesterol, No Free Sugar	6*	8†	3‡	11‡	3–4‡	5	. . .	. . .

* Inclusion of egg yolks is not recommended.

† Liquid vegetable oil and soft-type margarine, preferably made with liquid safflower oil or liquid corn oil, should be used.

‡ Amounts not restricted.

SUGGESTED MENU PATTERN

	Low Cholesterol	Low Cholesterol, No Free Sugar
Breakfast		
Fruit	1 serving	1 serving*
Cereal	1 serving	1 serving
Toast	1 slice	2 slices
Fat	2 teaspoons	2 teaspoons
Skim milk	1 cup	1 cup
Sugar, jelly	1 tablespoon	....
Beverage	1 cup	1 cup
Noon Meal		
Meat	3 ounces	3 ounces
Potato	1 serving	2 servings
Vegetable	1 serving	1 serving
Salad	1 serving	1 serving
Bread	1 slice	2 slices
Fat	3 teaspoons	3 teaspoons
Dessert	1 serving	2 servings*
Skim milk	....	1 cup
Sugar, jelly	1 tablespoon	....
Beverage	1 cup	1 cup
Evening Meal		
Meat	3 ounces	3 ounces
Potato	1 serving	2 servings
Vegetable	1 serving	1 serving
Salad	1 serving	1 serving
Bread	2 slices	2 slices
Fat	3 teaspoons	3 teaspoons
Dessert	1 serving	2 servings*
Skim milk	1 cup	1 cup
Sugar, jelly	1 tablespoon	....
Beverage	1 cup	1 cup

* Fresh or unsweetened fruits.

FOOD GROUPS

Low Cholesterol Diet

Allowed	Omitted

Beverage

Coffee, tea; carbonated beverage; cereal beverage

Meat

Meat, fish, or fowl, without visible fat or skin; cottage cheese and cheese made with low fat or skim milk; egg white, cholesterol-free egg powder. Bake, broil, pan broil, roast, stew, or fry in allowed oils if cooking temperature does not exceed 400 F	Fatty or heavily marbled meats, luncheon meats, frankfurters, sausages, brains, heart, kidney, liver, sweetbreads, tongue; duck, goose; crab and shrimp; egg yolks, foods containing egg yolks; cheese made with whole milk or cream; peanut butter

FOOD GROUPS

Low Cholesterol Diet

Allowed	Omitted

Fat

Listed in order of preference for increasing polyunsaturated fat content of diets:

Vegetable oils: safflower, corn, soybean, sesame, cottonseed

Margarine: liquid safflower oil margarine, liquid corn oil margarine

Nuts: walnuts, pecans, almonds

Salad dressings: mayonnaise, any other salad dressings except "Omitted"

(Omitted) Butter; completely hydrogenated margarines and vegetable shortenings, lard; peanut, olive, and coconut oils; avocado; bacon; cream, nondairy cream substitutes and whipped toppings, cream cheese; salad dressings with cream or cream cheese; nuts not "Allowed"; olives; fats from cooked meats

Milk

Skim milk, buttermilk; yogurt*

(Omitted) Whole milk, two percent milk, canned whole milk, chocolate milk; beverage mixes

Bread

Bread, quick breads, rolls, crackers except "Omitted"; cereals

(Omitted) Any with butter, cream, hydrogenated fat, dried egg, egg yolk, whole milk; butter or cheese crackers; commercially prepared baked goods, commercial mixes containing foods not "Allowed"

Potato and potato substitutes except "Omitted"; popcorn prepared with fats "Allowed"

(Omitted) Potato or other snack chips; buttered popcorn

FOOD GROUPS

Low Cholesterol Diet

Allowed	Omitted

Vegetable

Any

Fruit*

Any

Soup

Fat-free soups made from foods "Allowed"; packaged, dehydrated soups; broth, bouillon	Cream soups or any commercially prepared

Dessert*

Gelatin; sherbet; any cake, cookies, pastry, or pudding prepared with foods "Allowed"	Any with butter, chocolate, coconut, cream, dried eggs, egg yolk, whole milk, nuts not "Allowed"; commercially prepared mixes; ice cream, ice milk

Sweets*

Any except "Omitted"	Chocolate, coconut; candies made with chocolate, butter, cream, or coconut

FOOD GROUPS

Low Cholesterol Diet

Allowed	Omitted
Miscellaneous*	
Salt, spices, herbs, flavoring extracts; condiments; cocoa; pickles; vinegar, white sauce made with foods "Allowed"	Gravy, cream sauce; chocolate

*No Free Sugar Diet: omit foods with sugar added.

CARDIOVASCULAR DISEASES

SODIUM-RESTRICTED DIETS (20, 40, 90 Milliequivalents Sodium)

APPROXIMATE COMPOSITION (10 to 15% Variation)

Protein*	Fat	Carbohydrate	Calories	Sodium	Potassium	Fluid
gm	gm	gm		mEq	mEq	ml
70	95	230	2,055	Varies	80	2,000

*Value represents average amount of protein in general diet.

GENERAL INFORMATION

The physician may order diets with 20, 40, or 90 mEq of sodium. The diets containing 20 and 40 mEq of sodium are carefully controlled in order that the sodium content will vary only 10 to 15% from the prescribed level.

Some patients need a diet that is only moderately controlled in sodium (90 to 110 mEq). When such a mild restriction is indicated, the General Diet with no additional salt may be ordered. The following modifications are made: foods high in sodium are excluded and additional salt is not used at mealtime.

Diets containing less than 20 mEq of sodium may be ordered. The use of dialyzed or low sodium milk or the reduction of the amount of regular milk will be necessary if such diets are ordered.

Patients being instructed in the use of diets of 20 mEq of sodium or less are advised to check the sodium level of their local water supply. If the sodium level exceeds 1 mEq per quart, distilled water should be used. Chemically softened water should not be used on any sodium-restricted diet.

Protein Level of Sodium-Restricted Diets.   The Sodium-Restricted Diets are planned with 70 gm of protein. This level approximates the average amount of protein in the General Diet used in the hospital. Diets with higher levels of protein will contain more sodium because of the level of natural sodium in protein foods.

Protein Restrictions.   Diets with protein and sodium restrictions may be ordered by the physician. Appropriate diets are found in the section on "Dietary Program for Renal Diseases" (page 77).

SUGGESTED DAILY FOOD EXCHANGES (Mayo Clinic Food Exchange List, inside covers)

The Sodium-Restricted Diets are planned with the Mayo Clinic Food Exchange List. Servings of food exchanges are suggested in the table that follows. This table should be used only as a guide in planning the diets. Modifications within the prescribed diet may be made in order to adapt the diet to the normal dietary pattern of the hospital or the patient.

Sodium Level	Meat	Fat*	Milk	Bread	Vegetable	Fruit*	Dessert*	Sweets*
20 mEq	5	9	2	6	3–4	2–3	1	4
All foods are processed and prepared without salt								
40 mEq	5	9	2	6	3–4	2–3	1	4
May use 1/4 teaspoon of salt or salted fats								
All other foods processed or prepared without salt								
90–110 mEq	5	9	2	6	3–4	2–3	1	4
May use foods processed or prepared with a moderate amount of salt								
Omit use of salt at table and heavily salted foods								

*Amounts (unsalted) not restricted.

20 Milliequivalents Sodium.   All food included in the diet is prepared and processed without salt.

40 Milliequivalents Sodium.   All food included in the diet is prepared and processed without salt. The patient may choose to use either 1/4 teaspoon of salt at the table or salted fats.

90–110 Milliequivalents Sodium.   Foods processed or prepared with a moderate amount of salt may be used. Additional salt should not be used at the table on food which has been processed or prepared with salt or a sodium compound. Foods which have been preserved with a large amount of salt should not be used.

SUGGESTED MENU PATTERN

Breakfast		Noon Meal		Evening Meal	
Fruit	1 serving	Meat	2 ounces	Meat	2 ounces
Egg	1	Potato	1 serving	Potato	1 serving
Cereal	1 serving	Vegetable	1 serving	Vegetable	1 serving
Toast	1 slice	Salad	1 serving	Salad	1 serving
Fat	3 teaspoons	Bread	1 slice	Bread	1 slice
Sugar, jelly	2 tablespoons	Fat	3 teaspoons	Fat	3 teaspoons
Beverage	1 cup	Fruit	1 serving	Dessert	1 serving
		Sugar, jelly	1 tablespoon	Sugar, jelly	1 tablespoon
		Beverage	1 cup	Beverage	1 cup

FOOD GROUPS

Allowed	**Omitted**
	Food preserved or prepared with salt except where allowed on specific diets (General Information, page 22)

Beverages

Coffee, tea; carbonated beverages and mixes (if less than 1 mEq of sodium per 8 ounces); cereal beverage	

Meat

Unsalted meat, fowl, liver, heart, egg, cheese, or peanut butter; fish, fresh clams, oysters, or shrimp	Salted meat, fish, fowl, cheese, peanut butter; other organ meats; commercially frozen fish; other shellfish

Fat

Unsalted except "Omitted"; cream, 1/3 cup or less per day	Salted butter, margarine, salad dressings; bacon; olives; salted nuts

Milk

Any except "Omitted"; 1/3 cup of milk may be used in place of cream allowance	Buttermilk, commercial chocolate milk, beverage mixes; condensed milk

Bread

Salt-free bread, quick breads or rolls made with the following leavening agents: cream of tartar, potassium bicarbonate, sodium-free baking powder, yeast; unsalted crackers	Any made with salt, baking powder, or baking soda; commercially prepared mixes; self-rising flour
Unsalted cooked cereal; ready-to-eat cereals without salt	Instant, quick cooking, or ready-to-eat cereals with salt or sodium compound added*
Unsalted potato and potato substitutes	Commercially prepared mixes; potato chips; commercially frozen lima beans or peas; dried legumes; hominy; salted popcorn

Vegetable

Unsalted canned, cooked, fresh, or frozen except "Omitted"; no more than **one** serving daily of one of the following:	Any prepared with salt or sodium compounds

Artichokes	Collards
Beet greens	Dandelion greens
Beets	Kale
Carrots	Mustard greens
Celery	Spinach
Chard	White turnips

Fruit

Any canned, dried, fresh, or frozen

Allowed	Omitted

Soup
Unsalted soup or broth; cream soup made with milk allowance

Any other

Dessert
Unsalted cake and cookies made with the following leavening agents: cream of tartar, potassium bicarbonate, sodium-free baking powder; unsalted pie; sodium-free gelatin*; pudding or frozen dairy dessert when used as part of milk allowance

Desserts made with baking powder, baking soda, or salt; commercial dessert mixes

Sweets
Sugar; honey, jam, jelly, marmalade without a sodium preservative*; plain sugar candy

Chocolate and cream candies

Miscellaneous
Pepper, spices, and herbs except "Omitted"; flavoring extracts; bitter or sweet chocolate, cocoa powder; vinegar; unsalted white sauce; unsalted meat sauces

Salt or seasoning salts, mixed spices, dried celery products; bottled meat sauces, meat tenderizer, monosodium glutamate; pickles; milk chocolate, chocolate syrup, instant cocoa mix; gravy; regular baking powder, baking soda, salt substitutes unless approved by physician

*Consult list of ingredients on label or check with manufacturer.

DERMATITIS (ALLERGY)

COMMON IRRITANTS OMITTED

APPROXIMATE COMPOSITION (10 to 15% Variation)

Protein	Fat	Carbohydrate	Calories	Sodium	Potassium	Fluid
gm	gm	gm		mEq	mEq	ml
70	95	230	2,055	110	80	2,000

GENERAL INFORMATION

Sensitivity to food may be diagnosed by eliminating known or suspected food allergies. Frequently cited sources of food intolerances are listed below:

Meat Group
Cheese (except cottage cheese)
Corned beef
Eggs
Fish
Pork, fresh
Shellfish
Peanut butter

Fruit
Apple, fresh
Banana
Berries, fresh
Grapes
Pineapple
Rhubarb

Fat
Cream cheese
Nuts

Miscellaneous
Chocolate, cocoa; highly seasoned foods; strong spices; garlic

Vegetable
Corn
Tomatoes

The dietary program as outlined should be used for a limited time. Although the diet is nutritionally adequate, it may become monotonous if used indefinitely.

The diet is planned with the Mayo Clinic Food Exchange List. Servings of food exchanges are suggested in the following table. This table should be used only as a guide in planning the diets. Modifications within the prescribed dietary restriction may be made in order to adapt the diet to the normal dietary pattern of the hospital or the patient.

*SUGGESTED DAILY FOOD EXCHANGES** (Mayo Clinic Food Exchange
List, inside covers)

Meat	Fat	Milk	Bread	Vegetable	Fruit	Dessert	Sweets
5	9	2	6	3–4	2–3	1	4

*Amount not restricted.

SUGGESTED MENU PATTERN

Breakfast		**Noon Meal**		**Evening Meal**	
Fruit	1 serving	Meat	2 ounces	Meat	3 ounces
Cereal	1 serving	Potato	1 serving	Potato	1 serving
Toast	2 slices	Vegetable	1 serving	Vegetable	1 serving
Fat	3 teaspoons	Salad	1 serving	Salad	1 serving
Sugar, jelly	2 tablespoons	Bread	1 slice	Bread	1 slice
Beverage	1 cup	Fat	3 teaspoons	Butter	3 teaspoons
		Fruit	1 serving	Dessert	1 serving
		Milk	1 cup	Milk	1 cup
		Sugar, jelly	1 tablespoon	Sugar, jelly	1 tablespoon
		Beverage	1 cup	Beverage	1 cup

FOOD GROUPS

Allowed	Omitted
	Highly seasoned foods
Beverage	
Coffee, tea; carbonated beverage; cereal beverage	
Meat	
Any except "Omitted"; cottage cheese	Highly seasoned meats; fresh pork; fish, shellfish; eggs; other cheese; peanut butter
Fat	
Any except "Omitted"	Cream cheese; nuts; salad dressings with egg or cheese
Milk	
Milk, milk drinks	Chocolate milk, eggnog
Bread	
Any except "Omitted"	Commercially prepared mixes; any with eggs or nuts; corn
Vegetable	
Any except "Omitted"	Tomatoes
Fruit	
Any except "Omitted"	Banana, fresh apple or berries, grapes, pineapple, rhubarb
Soup	
Any except "Omitted"	Any with corn, tomatoes, shellfish
Dessert	
Any except "Omitted"	Any with chocolate, cocoa, eggs, nuts, or "Omitted" fruits; commercially prepared mixes
Sweets	
Any except "Omitted"	Jelly, jam, marmalade with "Omitted" fruits; candy with chocolate, eggs, nuts, or "Omitted" fruits
Miscellaneous	
Salt; spices, herbs except "Omitted"; vinegar; pickles; gravy, white sauce	Garlic; strong spices; chocolate, cocoa

PENICILLIN ELIMINATION DIET

Food contaminants may cause allergic reactions. The presence of penicillin in milk and milk products should be considered as a possible cause of allergic reactions.

A general diet is served with the exception of these foods or any foods prepared with these products:

Fresh whole milk	Cream
Skim milk	Cheese
Buttermilk	Cottage cheese

The following foods may be used:

Dry powdered milk (whole or skim)
Condensed milk
Ice cream, sherbet, fruit ice
Butter

DIABETES

DIABETIC DIETS

NUTRITIONAL ADEQUACY

Diets of less than 1,000 calories may be nutritionally inadequate. The physician may wish to prescribe vitamin and mineral supplements (page 134). All other diets are nutritionally adequate according to the Recommended Daily Dietary Allowances of the National Research Council (page 130).

APPROXIMATE COMPOSITION (10 to 15% Variation)

Calories	Protein	Fat	Carbohydrate	Sodium*	Potassium	Fluid
	gm	gm	gm	mEq	mEq	ml
800	60	30	80	55	70	1,800
1,000	70	40	90	65	75	1,800
1,200	75	50	120	85	85	1,900
1,400	75	70	120	85	85	1,900
1,600	80	80	145	100	90	2,000
1,800	80	90	170	120	95	2,000
2,000	90	100	185	130	95	2,000
2,200	100	110	210	135	110	2,300
2,400	110	120	220	145	115	2,300
2,600	115	135	230	155	120	2,600
2,800	125	140	260	170	135	2,800
3,000	130	150	285	185	140	2,800

*Value is for average amount of salt used in preparation of food; salt added to food at the table is not calculated.

GENERAL INFORMATION

The diabetic diets are planned according to the Mayo Clinic Food Exchange Lists (inside covers). The Mayo Clinic Food Exchange List was developed from a method adopted by the American Diabetes Association, United States Public Health Service, and the American Dietetic Association. Patterns have been established for diets from 800 to 3,000 calories. Diabetic diets of more than 3,000 calories are available on request. Bedtime feedings are planned routinely for all diabetic diets.

The diet is calculated according to the need of the patient for calories, protein, fat, and carbohydrate, based on age, sex, height, ideal weight, and activity. Calories from fat range from 35 to 45% of the total calories. The diabetic diet may be ordered as either "weighed" or "not weighed."

The dietitian will calculate the carbohydrate value of all food refused by diabetic patients. Food replacement is given to patients receiving insulin or an oral agent when the carbohydrate value of food refused exceeds 25 gm per meal.

Diabetic diets ordered with additional dietary modifications follow the general pattern of the standard diabetic diets. Such diets are planned according to the Mayo Clinic Food Exchange List.

The dietary program for diabetic patients after surgical treatment follows the general pattern of the surgical dietary regimen. With the exception of sugar, foods allowed in the clear liquid, full liquid, and soft diets are served. The patient progresses to the prescribed diabetic diet as soon as it can be tolerated.

METHOD FOR DETERMINING CALORIE LEVEL

The physician prescribes the calorie level of the diet by selecting percentage increment in calories above the basal requirements. The following allowances frequently are used in determining the total calorie level:

50 to 80%	Heavy work
20 to 40%	Moderate work
10 to 20%	Light work

The basal calorie requirements of the patient are calculated according to the directions of the food nomogram (page 160). The calorie level of the diet is determined primarily by the ideal weight or desired weight of the patient. Adjustments in the diet should be made as fluctuations occur in the maintenance of the desired weight.

A sample determination of a diabetic diet follows:

Patient: 40-year-old man; 5 feet 8 inches tall; 155 pounds (ideal weight) ; office worker

	Calories
Basal calorie requirement	1,660
40% increment of basal calorie requirement	664
Total	2,324
Calorie level of diabetic diet	2,400

ADMISSION DIET FOR PATIENTS WITH DIABETES

The 1,800 calorie diabetic diet is served routinely to diabetic patients admitted to the hospital without a diet prescription. This diet should be used temporarily until the appropriate diet has been prescribed by the physician.

SUGGESTED MENU PATTERN (Mayo Clinic Food Exchange List, inside covers)

1,800 Calorie Diabetic Admission Diet

Breakfast

Fruit	1 exchange
Meat	1 exchange
Bread	2 exchanges
Fat	2 exchanges
Beverage	

Noon Meal

Meat	3 exchanges
Bread	2 exchanges
Fat	2 exchanges
Vegetable A	1 exchange
Fruit	1 exchange
Milk	1 exchange
Beverage	

Evening Meal

Meat	3 exchanges
Bread	2 exchanges
Fat	2 exchanges
Vegetable A	1 exchange
Vegetable B	1 exchange
Fruit	1 exchange
Beverage	

Bedtime

Milk	1 exchange
Bread	2 exchanges
Fat	1 exchange

SUGGESTED SERVINGS OF FOOD EXCHANGES

Servings of food exchanges from the Mayo Clinic Food Exchange List for each diabetic diet are suggested in the following table. This table should be used only as a guide in planning the diets. Modifications within the prescribed dietary restrictions may be made in order to adapt the diet to the normal dietary pattern of the hospital or the patient.

SUGGESTED DAILY FOOD EXCHANGES (Mayo Clinic Food Exchange List, inside covers)

Calories	Meat	Fat	Milk	Bread	Vegetable B*	Fruit
800	6	. . .	2 (skim)	1	1	3
1,000	7	1	2 (skim)	2	1	3
1,200	7	3	2 (skim)	4	1	3
1,400	7	3	2	4	1	3
1,600	7	5	2	6	1	3
1,800	7	7	2	8	1	3
2,000	8	8	2	9	1	3
2,200	8	8	3	9	1	4
2,400	9	9	3	10	1	4
2,600	9	10	4	10	1	4
2,800	10	10	4	11	1	5
3,000	10	12	4	13	1	5

*Vegetable A Food Group may be included in ordinary amounts with each meal.

SUGGESTED MENU PATTERN

Food exchanges may be served as suggested in the following table. The table should be used only as a guide in planning the diets. Modifications within the prescribed dietary restrictions may be made in order to adapt the diet to the normal dietary pattern of the hospital or the patient.

FOODS AS DESIRED

An exchange is not necessary for the following foods because they do not contain an appreciable amount of protein, fat, or carbohydrate.

Bouillon, broth, or consommé, fat free
Catsup (1 tbsp or 15 gm)
Chives
Coffee
Cranberries (unsweetened)
Cress
Decaffeinated coffee
Endive
Flavoring extracts
Gelatin, unsweetened (flavored or unflavored)
Herbs
Horseradish

Lemon juice
Lime juice
Meat sauces (prepared without sugar)
Mustard
Parsley
Pepper
Pickles (dill or sour)
Rhubarb (unsweetened)
Salt
Spices
Tea
Vinegar

DIABETIC MENU PATTERNS

Calories	800	1,000	1,200	1,400	1,600	1,800	2,000	2,200	2,400	2,600	2,800	3,000
Food Exchanges						Number of Exchanges						
Breakfast												
Fruit	1	1	1	1	1	1	1	1	1	1	1	1
Meat	1	1	1	1	1	1	1	1	2	2	2	2
Bread	1	1	1	1	1	2	2	2	2	2	3	3
Fat	...	1	1	1	1	2	2	2	2	3	3	3
Milk*	...	...	...	...	...	...	...	1	1	1	1	1
Noon Meal												
Meat	2	3	3	3	3	3	3	3	3	3	3	3
Bread	...	...	1	1	2	2	2	2	3	3	3	4
Fat	...	...	1	1	2	2	2	2	3	3	3	4
Vegetable A	1	1	1	1	1	1	1	1	1	1	1	1
Fruit	1	1	1	1	1	1	1	2	2	2	2	2
Milk*	1†	1†	1†	1	1	1	1	1	1	1	1	1
Evening Meal												
Meat	3	3	3	3	3	3	3	3	3	3	3	3
Bread	...	...	1	1	2	2	3	3	3	3	3	4
Fat	...	...	1	1	2	2	3	3	3	3	3	4
Vegetable A	1	1	1	1	1	1	1	1	1	1	1	1
Vegetable B	1	1	1	1	1	1	1	1	1	1	1	1
Fruit	1	1	1	1	1	1	1	1	1	1	2	2
Milk*	...	...	...	...	...	...	...	...	...	1	1	1
Bedtime												
Milk*	1†	1†	1†	1	1	1	1	1	1	1	1	1
Bread	...	1	1	1	1	2	2	2	2	2	2	2
Fat	...	...	...	...	...	1	1	1	1	1	1	1
Meat	...	...	...	...	...	...	1	1	1	1	2	2

*Milk may be distributed as desired.
†Skim milk.

GASTROINTESTINAL DISORDERS

BLAND DIET

APPROXIMATE COMPOSITION (10 to 15% Variation)

Protein	Fat	Carbohydrate	Calories	Sodium*	Potassium	Fluid
gm	gm	gm		mEq	mEq	ml
70	95	230	2,055	110	80	2,000

*Value is for average amount of salt used in preparation of food; salt added to food at the table is not calculated.

GENERAL INFORMATION

The Bland Diet is ordered when conservative dietary features are indicated as part of the management of gastrointestinal disorders. Although the diet should be individualized according to food intolerances, certain condiments and foods that are highly seasoned usually are eliminated. Foods are included that are moderately low in connective tissue and fiber. Emphasis is placed on a normal diet pattern.

The Bland Diet is planned with the Mayo Clinic Food Exchange List. Servings of food exchanges that will provide a nutritionally adequate diet are suggested in the following table. This table should be used only as a guide in planning the diets. Modifications within the prescribed dietary restrictions may be made in order to adapt the diet to the normal dietary pattern of the hospital or the patient.

SUGGESTED DAILY FOOD EXCHANGES* (Mayo Clinic Food Exchange List, inside covers)

Meat	Fat	Milk	Bread	Vegetable	Fruit	Dessert	Sweets
5	9	2	6	3–4	2–3	1	4

*Amounts not restricted.

SUGGESTED MENU PATTERN

Breakfast		Noon Meal		Evening Meal	
Fruit	1 serving	Meat	2 ounces	Meat	2 ounces
Egg	1	Potato	1 serving	Potato	1 serving
Cereal	1 serving	Vegetable	1 serving	Vegetable	1 serving
Toast	1 slice	Salad	1 serving	Salad	1 serving
Fat	3 teaspoons	Bread	1 slice	Bread	1 slice
Sugar, jelly	2 tablespoons	Fat	3 teaspoons	Fat	3 teaspoons
Beverage	1 cup	Fruit	1 serving	Milk	1 cup
		Milk	1 cup	Dessert	1 serving
		Sugar, jelly	1 tablespoon	Sugar, jelly	1 tablespoon
		Beverage	1 cup	Beverage	1 cup

FOOD GROUPS

Allowed	Omitted
	Fried and highly seasoned foods
Beverage	
Coffee, tea; carbonated beverage; cereal beverage	
Meat	
Meat, fish, or fowl; egg; cottage cheese, mild cheese used as flavoring; cream style peanut butter	Fried; highly seasoned meats or fish; other cheese
Fat	
Any except "Omitted"	Avocado; nuts; olives; highly seasoned salad dressings
Milk	
Milk, milk drinks	
Bread	
Refined wheat, graham, or rye bread, rolls, quick breads, or crackers	Any with whole grain flour, bran, seeds, or nuts
Refined cereals — cooked or ready to eat	Whole grain or bran cereals
Potato or potato substitutes except "Omitted"; puréed corn, lima beans, peas; hominy grits	Whole grain rice; dried legumes; popcorn; potato chips, fried potatoes
Vegetable	
Canned or cooked mild-flavored vegetables without seeds or coarse fiber; lettuce, tomatoes (no seeds or skin)	Raw except "Allowed"; strong flavored
Fruit	
Canned or cooked, fresh or frozen fruit without seeds, tough skin, or membrane; fruit juice	Any other
Soup	
Broth, bouillon, or cream soup with "Allowed" vegetables; commercial, as tolerated	Any other
Dessert	
Any except "Omitted"	Any with coconut, nuts, or "Omitted" fruits
Sweets	
Any except "Omitted"	Jam, marmalade; candy with coconut, nuts, or "Omitted" fruits
Miscellaneous	
Salt; spices and herbs except "Omitted"; condiments, as tolerated; chocolate, cocoa; gravy, white sauce; vinegar	Pepper, chili powder, cloves, seed spices, garlic; pickles

DIET FOR GASTRIC OBSTRUCTION

NUTRITIONAL ADEQUACY

The diet for gastric obstruction does not meet the Recommended Daily Dietary Allowances of the National Research Council for vitamins and minerals. The physician may wish to prescribe supplements.

APPROXIMATE COMPOSITION (10 to 15% Variation)

Protein	Fat	Carbohydrate	Calories	Sodium*	Potassium	Fluid
gm	gm	gm		mEq	mEq	ml
65	90	245	2,050	90	80	2,400

*Value is for average amount of salt used in preparation of food; salt added to food at the table is not calculated.

GENERAL INFORMATION

The diet may be ordered in cases of gastric retention caused by an obstructive lesion at the outlet of the stomach. Small meals of liquids are served every 2 hours from 8 a.m. to 8 p.m. Foods that stimulate secretion of gastric acid such as coffee, tea, meat extracts, and spices are eliminated from the diet. When removal of food through a tube by suction is necessary, only foods that liquefy at body temperature are allowed.

The diet is planned with the Mayo Clinic Food Exchange List. High calorie foods should be served at between-meal feedings to provide additional calories. Servings of food exchanges that may be included in the diet are suggested in the following table. This table should be used only as a guide in planning the diets. Modifications within the prescribed dietary restriction may be made in order to adapt the diet to the dietary pattern of the hospital or the patient.

SUGGESTED DAILY FOOD EXCHANGES* (Mayo Clinic Food Exchange List, inside covers)

Egg	Fat	Milk	Cereal	Vegetable	Fruit	Dessert	Sweets
1⁺	3	5	1	1	2	2	1

*As tolerated.
⁺Eggnog or custard.

SUGGESTED MENU PATTERN

Breakfast

Juice	1 serving
Cereal gruel	1 serving
Half and half	1/3 cup
Sugar	1 tablespoon
Eeverage	1 cup

10 a. m.

Milk drink	1 cup

Noon Meal

Cream soup, strained	1 serving
Dessert	1 serving
Milk	1/2 cup
Beverage	1 cup

2 p. m.

Milk drink	1 cup

4 p. m.

Milk	1 cup

Evening Meal

Cream soup, strained	1 serving
Fruit juice	1 serving
Dessert	1 serving
Milk	1/2 cup
Beverage	1 cup

8 p. m.

Milk drink	1 cup

FOOD GROUPS

Allowed: Only Foods Listed

Beverage
Cereal beverage; decaffeinated coffee

Egg
Dried egg powder in milk drinks or custard

Fat
Butter, margarine; half and half

Bread
Cereal gruel

Milk
Milk, milk drinks

Vegetable
Mild-flavored juice or purée in soup

Fruit
Fruit juice, strained

Soup
Cream soup, strained

Dessert
Custard, pudding, ice cream, sherbet — all without coconut, nuts, or whole fruit

Sweets
Sugar

Miscellaneous
Salt; cocoa, chocolate

DIETS FOR ULCERS

APPROXIMATE COMPOSITION (10 to 15% Variation)

Diet	Protein gm	Fat gm	Carbohydrate gm	Calories	Sodium* mEq	Potassium mEq	Fluid ml
Milk Regimen	50	75	90	1,235	40	70	1,600
Hospital Strict Ulcer	90	100	210	2,100	105	95	2,600
Convalescent Patient							
Strict Ulcer	95	110	210	2,210	110	105	2,600
Liberal Ulcer	90	110	220	2,230	120	100	2,600

*Value is for average amount of salt used in preparation of food; salt added to food at the table is not calculated.

GENERAL PRINCIPLES

General principles used in planning ulcer diets have been based on unverified impressions and traditional food intolerances. Chemical studies have not shown any proved value of usual diet restrictions. Nevertheless, diet therapy for patients who have peptic ulcer remains a part of the medical treatment. The diet regimen is designed to inhibit acid output and to neutralize any gastric secretions. In addition, the diet should help to relieve pain caused by ulcers and to promote healing.

The diets omit foods frequently indicated as causing gastric irritation by most patients with ulcers, although these foods may be satisfactory for some individuals. Foods that have a slightly stimulating effect on gastric acid secretion or acid-buffering qualities or both are included.

The physician should order a diet in accordance with the severity of the ulcer symptoms. Intermeal feedings of allowed foods are included with each diet. Antacids are added on the direction of the physician.

DESCRIPTION OF DIETARY REGIMENS

The regimens for patients with gastrointestinal disturbances are as follows:

Milk Regimen.   During the acute stages of ulcer symptoms, hourly feedings of 4 ounces of milk may be served between 7:30 a.m. and 9:30 p.m. Whole milk, skim milk, or milk beverages may be used. For obese patients, skim milk should be ordered.

This regimen should be used for a limited time, since most nutrients provided by this diet are less than the recommended dietary allowances for adults.

Hospital Strict Ulcer Diet.   Three small meals consisting of liquid, soft, and low fiber foods may be ordered as a supplement to hourly feedings. Meat products are not permitted; fruit juices and puréed fruits and vegetables are allowed. The fiber content is negligible.

Strict Ulcer Diet for Convalescent Patients.   Three meals consisting of soft and low fiber foods are allowed on this diet. Meats, fish, or fowl and whole-cooked fruits and vegetables are allowed. Hourly supplements of allowed foods should be included.

Liberal Ulcer Diet for Convalescent Patients.   Most foods in the normal diet may be used in this liberal ulcer diet. Foods that are highly seasoned or that may cause excessive stimulation of gastric secretion are eliminated. The diet may contain a moderate amount of fiber, depending on individual tolerance. Between-meal feedings of allowed foods should be included.

Dietary regimens for ulcers are planned with the Mayo Clinic Food Exchange List. Servings of food exchanges that may be included in the diet are suggested in the following table. This table should be used only as a guide in planning the diets. Modifications within the prescribed dietary restrictions may be made in order to adapt the diet to the normal dietary pattern of the hospital or the patient. The amount of fat in the diet does not exceed 45% of the calories.

SUGGESTED DAILY FOOD EXCHANGES (Mayo Clinic Food Exchange List, inside covers)

Diet	Milk	Meat	Fat	Bread	Vegetable	Fruit	Dessert	Sweets
Milk Regimen	7 1/2	...	...	...	...	...	...	...
Hospital Strict Ulcer	6	4*	3	4	2	2	1	1
Convalescent Patient								
Strict Ulcer	6	5	3	4	3	2	1	1
Liberal Ulcer	5	5	5	6	4	2	1	1

*No meat, fish, or fowl allowed; see page 42 for meat substitutes.

Hospital Strict Ulcer Diet

NUTRITIONAL ADEQUACY

The Hospital Strict Ulcer Diet does not meet the recommended levels for vitamins and minerals according to the Recommended Daily Dietary Allowances of the National Research Council. The physician may wish to order vitamin and mineral supplements for patients who remain on the diet for any extended time.

GENERAL INFORMATION

The Hospital Strict Ulcer Diet is planned for a patient who is confined to the hospital due to severity of ulcer symptoms.

Three small meals of soft and low fiber foods are served. Four ounces of milk or milk beverage is given hourly as intermeal and before-bedtime feedings.

SUGGESTED MENU PATTERN (Four ounces of milk hourly between meals until bedtime)

Breakfast		Noon Meal		Evening Meal	
Fruit	1 serving	Meat substitute*	1	Meat substitute*	2
Egg	1	Vegetable	1 serving	Potato	1 serving
Toast	1 slice	Bread	1 slice	Vegetable	1 serving
Fat	1 teaspoon	Fat	1 teaspoon	Bread	1 slice
Sugar	1 teaspoon	Fruit	1 serving	Fat	1 teaspoon
Beverage	1 cup	Sugar	1 teaspoon	Dessert	1 serving
		Beverage	1 cup	Sugar	1 teaspoon
				Beverage	1 cup

*See page 42 for meat substitute.

FOOD GROUPS

Allowed	Omitted
	Fried and highly seasoned foods
Beverage	
Cereal beverages; decaffeinated coffee	
Meat substitutes	
Egg; cottage cheese, mild cheese used as flavoring; cream style peanut butter	Meat, fish, or fowl; other cheese
Fat	
Any except "Omitted"	Avocado; bacon; nuts; olives; highly seasoned salad dressings
Milk	
Milk, milk drinks	
Bread	
Refined wheat or rye bread, rolls, or crackers	Any with graham or whole grain flour, bran, seeds, or nuts; quick breads
Refined cereals — cooked or ready to eat	Whole grain or bran cereals
Potato and potato substitutes except "Omitted"; puréed corn, lima beans, peas; hominy grits	Whole grain rice; dried legumes; popcorn; potato chips, fried potatoes
Vegetable	
Mild-flavored vegetables: purée or juice	Any other
Fruit	
Purée or juice	Any other
Soup	
Cream soup with vegetable purée	Broth, bouillon; commercial soups
Dessert	
Any except "Omitted"	Any with coconut, nuts, or whole fruit; pastries
Sweets	
Any except "Omitted"	Jam, marmalade; candy with coconut, nuts, or fruits
Miscellaneous	
Salt, spices and herbs except "Omitted"; chocolate, cocoa; white sauce	Pepper, chili powder, cloves, seed spices; condiments; pickles; gravy

Strict Ulcer Diet for Convalescent Patients

GENERAL INFORMATION

The Strict Ulcer Diet for Convalescent Patients is ordered for patients whose activities are restricted because of ulcer symptoms. This diet also is ordered for ambulatory patients when any ulcer symptoms occur. The physician may indicate instructions for a patient for both the strict and the liberal ulcer diets.

Meat, fish, or fowl is included in this diet. Certain whole fruits and vegetables are permitted. The meals are supplemented with 4 ounces of milk or milk beverage hourly between meals until bedtime.

SUGGESTED MENU PATTERN   (Four ounces of milk
hourly between meals until bedtime)

Breakfast		Noon Meal		Evening Meal	
Fruit	1 serving	Meat	2 ounces	Meat	2 ounces
Egg	1	Potato	1 serving	Potato	1 serving
Toast	1 slice	Vegetable	1 serving	Vegetable	1 serving
Fat	1 teaspoon	Bread	1 slice	Salad	1 serving
Sugar	1 teaspoon	Fat	1 teaspoon	Fat	1 teaspoon
Beverage	1 cup	Fruit	1 serving	Dessert	1 serving
		Sugar	1 teaspoon	Sugar	1 teaspoon
		Beverage	1 cup	Beverage	1 cup

FOOD GROUPS

Allowed	Omitted
	Fried and highly seasoned foods
Beverage	
Cereal beverage; decaffeinated coffee	Carbonated beverage, coffee, tea
Meat	
Meat, fish, or fowl; egg; cottage cheese, mild cheese used as flavoring; cream style peanut butter	Fried; preserved meats or fish; other cheese
Fat	
Any except "Omitted"	Avocado; bacon; nuts; olives; highly seasoned salad dressings
Milk	
Milk, milk drinks	
Bread	
Refined wheat or rye bread, rolls, or crackers; quick breads as tolerated	Any with graham or whole grain flour, bran, seeds, or nuts
Refined cereals— cooked or ready to eat	Whole grain or bran cereals
Potato and potato substitutes except "Omitted"; puréed corn, lima beans, peas; hominy grits	Whole grain rice; dried legumes; popcorn; potato chips, fried potatoes
Vegetable	
Canned or cooked mild-flavored vegetables without seeds or coarse fiber; lettuce, tomatoes (no seeds or skin)	Any other raw; strong flavored
Fruit	
Canned or cooked fruits without seeds or tough skin; fruit juice; banana, citrus fruit without membrane	Any other
Soup	
Cream soup with "Allowed" vegetables	Broth, bouillon; commercial soups
Dessert	
Any except "Omitted"	Any with coconut, nuts, or "Omitted" fruits; pastries
Sweets	
Any except "Omitted"	Jam, marmalade; candy with coconut, nuts, or "Omitted" fruits
Miscellaneous	
Salt, spices, and herbs except "Omitted"; chocolate, cocoa; vinegar; white sauce	Chili powder, cloves, pepper, seed spices; condiments; pickles; gravy

Liberal Ulcer Diet for Convalescent Patients

GENERAL INFORMATION

The Liberal Ulcer Diet for Convalescent Patients is ordered for hospitalized or ambulatory patients who are not having ulcer symptoms. The diet for a patient free of ulcer symptoms may include most foods in a normal diet. Foods that are highly seasoned or cause excessive stimulation of gastric secretion are eliminated. The diet is planned with between-meal feedings of allowed foods.

SUGGESTED MENU PATTERN (Eight ounces of milk between each meal and at bedtime)

Breakfast		Noon Meal		Evening Meal	
Fruit	1 serving	Meat	2 ounces	Meat	2 ounces
Egg	1	Potato	1 serving	Potato	1 serving
Cereal	1 serving	Vegetable	1 serving	Vegetable	1 serving
Toast	1 slice	Salad	1 serving	Bread	1 slice
Fat	3 teaspoons	Bread	1 slice	Fat	1 teaspoon
Sugar, jelly	1 teaspoon	Fat	1 teaspoon	Dessert	1 serving
Beverage	1 cup	Fruit	1 serving	Milk	1 cup
		Milk	1 cup	Sugar	1 teaspoon
		Sugar	1 teaspoon	Beverage	1 cup
		Beverage	1 cup		

FOOD GROUPS

Allowed	Omitted
Beverage Tea; cereal beverage; decaffeinated coffee	*Highly seasoned foods* Carbonated beverage; coffee (unless approved by physician)
Meat Meat, fish, or fowl; preserved meats or fish, as tolerated Egg; cottage cheese, cheese; cream style peanut butter	Meat or cheese with "Omitted" seasonings
Fat Any except "Omitted"	Olives; nuts; highly seasoned salad dressings
Milk Milk, milk drinks	
Bread Refined wheat, graham, or rye bread, rolls, or crackers Refined cereals — cooked or ready to eat Potato and potato substitutes except "Omitted"; puréed corn; tender lima beans and peas	Any with whole grain flour, bran, seeds, or nuts Whole grain or bran cereals Whole grain rice; dried legumes; popcorn
Vegetable Canned, cooked, frozen, or fresh mild-flavored vegetables without seeds, skins, or coarse fiber	Strong flavored
Fruit Canned, cooked, fresh, or frozen fruits without seeds, tough skin, or membrane; fruit juice	Any other
Soup Cream soup with "Allowed" vegetables	Broth, bouillon; commercial soups
Dessert Any except "Omitted"	Any with coconut, nuts, or "Omitted" fruits
Sweets Any except "Omitted"	Jam, marmalade; candy with coconut, nuts, or "Omitted" fruits
Miscellaneous Salt, spices, and herbs except "Omitted"; chocolate, cocoa; vinegar; white sauce	Chili powder, cloves, pepper, seed spices, garlic; gravy; pickles

DIETS FOR CHRONIC AND INFLAMMATORY INTESTINAL DISORDERS

Foundation Diet and Full Diet

NUTRITIONAL ADEQUACY

The Foundation Diet does not meet the Recommended Daily Dietary Allowances of the National Research Council. The physician may wish to order vitamin and mineral supplements. The Full Diet meets the recommended nutrient levels.

APPROXIMATE COMPOSITION (10 to 15% Variation)

Diet	Protein gm	Fat gm	Carbohydrate gm	Calories	Sodium* mEq	Potassium mEq	Fluid ml
Foundation	95	120	235	2,400	130	65	1,300
Full	120	140	315	3,000	155	110	2,300

*Value is for average amount of salt used in preparation of food; salt added to food at the table is not calculated.

GENERAL INFORMATION

The physician may order the Foundation Diet or the Full Diet for management of either chronic ulcerative colitis or regional enteritis. The choice of diet should be based on the severity of symptoms.

Foundation Diet.   This diet may be ordered for patients with severe characteristic symptoms. Protein and calories are slightly higher than in the regular diet for adults. The diet is low in residue; milk, fruits, and vegetables are omitted. When symptoms become less severe, the Full Diet may be ordered. The Full Diet may be given immediately or in a gradual stepwise fashion. See Advancement to Full Diet, page 51.

Full Diet.   This diet may be ordered for patients with less severe characteristic symptoms. The diet is moderately low in residue; milk, fruits, and vegetables are included. Because loss of weight is a frequent symptom, calories should be increased with high calorie foods as tolerated by the patient. The level of protein is approximately 80% higher than suggested for the average adult, and calories are increased approximately 80% above basal calorie requirements. The diet may be modified to a higher or lower level of either nutrient if the physician desires.

The diets are planned with the Mayo Clinic Food Exchange List. Servings of food exchanges are suggested in the following table. This table should be used only as a guide in planning the diets. Modifications within the prescribed dietary restrictions may be made in order to adapt the diet to the normal dietary pattern of the hospital or the patient.

SUGGESTED DAILY FOOD EXCHANGES* (Mayo Clinic Food Exchange List, inside covers)

Diet	Meat	Fat	Milk	Bread	Vegetable	Fruit	Dessert	Sweets
Foundation	10	12	...†	9	...	...	2	4
Full	10	9	3	9	3	2	2	6

*Amounts not restricted.
†A small amount of milk may be used in cooking (1/2 cup or less).

SUGGESTED MENU PATTERNS

	Foundation Diet	**Full Diet**
Breakfast		
Fruit	...	1 serving
Egg	1	1
Cereal	1 serving	1 serving
Toast	2 slices	2 slices
Fat	4 teaspoons	3 teaspoons
Milk	...	1 cup
Sugar, jelly	2 tablespoons	2 tablespoons
Beverage	1 cup	1 cup
Noon Meal		
Meat	4 ounces	4 ounces
Potato	1 serving	1 serving
Vegetable	...	1 serving
Salad	...	1 serving
Bread	2 slices	2 slices
Fat	4 teaspoons	3 teaspoons
Dessert	1 serving	1 serving
Milk	...	1 cup
Sugar, jelly	1 tablespoon	2 tablespoons
Beverage	1 cup	1 cup
Evening Meal		
Meat	5 ounces	5 ounces
Potato	1 serving	1 serving
Vegetable	...	1 serving
Salad	...	1 serving
Bread	2 slices	2 slices
Fat	4 teaspoons	3 teaspoons
Dessert	1 serving	1 serving
Milk	...	1 cup
Sugar, jelly	1 tablespoon	2 tablespoons
Beverage	1 cup	1 cup

Foundation Diet

FOOD GROUPS

Allowed	Omitted
Beverage	
Coffee, tea; carbonated beverage; cereal beverage	
Meat	
Meat, fish, or fowl; egg; cheese; cream style peanut butter	
Fat	
Any except "Omitted"	Avocado; nuts; olives; salad dressings
Milk	
A small amount used in cooking (1/2 cup or less)	Milk, milk drinks
Bread	
Refined wheat or rye bread, quick breads, rolls, or crackers	Any with graham, or whole grain flour, bran, seeds, or nuts
Refined cereals—cooked or ready to eat	Whole grain or bran cereals
Potato and potato substitutes except "Omitted"; hominy grits	Whole grain rice; dried legumes; popcorn; corn, lima beans, peas
Vegetable	
None	All
Fruit	
None	All
Soup	
Bouillon, broth	Any except "Allowed"
Dessert	
Any except "Omitted"; puddings and ice cream within milk allowance	Any with coconut, nuts, or fruits
Sweets	
Any except "Omitted"	Jam, marmalade; candy with coconut, nuts, or fruit
Miscellaneous	
Salt, spices, and herbs except "Omitted"; chocolate; gravy, white sauce; vinegar	Garlic; pickles; cocoa

ADVANCEMENT TO FULL DIET

In most cases, the patient on a Foundation Diet may progress directly to the Full Diet when characteristic symptoms decrease in severity. If the physician desires a slower progression, he may order a stepwise addition of the following foods to be made every 2 days. If so, the addition at which the advancement is to start should be specified:

Addition 1. Banana, orange juice
Addition 2. Mild-flavored vegetables (puréed or juice)
Addition 3. Boiled milk
Addition 4. Milk (not boiled)
Addition 5. Fruit: Canned or cooked without seeds or tough skin; citrus fruits without membranes
Addition 6. Mild-flavored vegetable: Canned or cooked without seeds or coarse fiber
Addition 7. Lettuce; plain salad dressings

Full Diet

FOOD GROUPS

Allowed	Omitted
Beverage	
Coffee, tea; carbonated beverage; cereal beverage	
Meat	
Meat, fish, or fowl; egg; cheese; cream style peanut butter	
Fat	
Any except "Omitted"	Avocado; nuts; olives
Milk	
Milk, milk drinks	
Bread	
Refined wheat or rye bread, rolls, or crackers; quick breads	Any with graham or whole grain flour, bran, seeds, or nuts
Refined cereals—cooked or ready to eat	Whole grain or bran cereals
Potato and potato substitutes except "Omitted"; puréed corn, lima beans, peas; hominy grits	Whole grain rice; dried legumes; popcorn
Vegetable	
Canned or cooked mild-flavored vegetables without seeds or coarse fiber; lettuce, tomato (no seeds or skins)	Strong flavored

Allowed	Omitted
Fruit	
Canned, or cooked without seeds or tough skin; fruit juice; banana, citrus fruit without membrane	Any other; prunes
Soup	
Broth, bouillon, cream soup with "Allowed" vegetables	Any except "Allowed"
Dessert	
Any except "Omitted"	Any with coconut, nuts, or "Omitted" fruits
Sweets	
Any except "Omitted"	Jam, marmalade; candy with coconut, nuts, or "Omitted" fruits
Miscellaneous	
Salt, spices, and herbs except "Omitted"; cocoa; condiments; gravy, white sauce; vinegar	Garlic; pickles

DIET FOR NONTROPICAL SPRUE

Gluten-Restricted Diet

NUTRITIONAL ADEQUACY

The Gluten-Restricted Diet is nutritionally adequate according to the Recommended Daily Dietary Allowances of the National Research Council. The physician may wish to order vitamin and mineral supplements.

APPROXIMATE COMPOSITION (10 to 15% Variation)

Protein	Fat	Carbohydrate	Calories	Sodium*	Potassium	Fluid
gm	gm	gm		mEq	mEq	ml
70	95	230	2,055	110	80	2,000

*Value is for average amount of salt used in preparation of food; salt added to food at the table is not calculated.

GENERAL INFORMATION

The Gluten-Restricted Diet may be ordered for patients with nontropical sprue (celiac sprue or gluten-induced sprue). Gluten is removed from the diet by eliminating all foods prepared with wheat, rye, oats, barley, and buckwheat. Many packaged and processed foods should be omitted. They may contain gluten in combination with stabilizers. The diet is not restricted in fat or fiber unless so specified by the physician.

The diet is planned with the Mayo Clinic Food Exchange List. Servings of daily food exchanges are suggested in the table that follows. This table should be used only as a guide in planning the diet. Modifications within the prescribed dietary restrictions may be made in order to adapt the diet to the normal dietary pattern of the hospital or the patient.

SUGGESTED DAILY FOOD EXCHANGES* (Mayo Clinic Food Exchange List, inside covers)

Meat	Fat	Milk	Bread	Vegetable	Fruit	Dessert	Sweets
5	9	2	6†	3–4	2–3	1	4

*Amounts not restricted.
†Note limitations listed on page 54.

SUGGESTED MENU PATTERN

Breakfast		Noon Meal		Evening Meal	
Fruit	1 serving	Meat	2 ounces	Meat	2 ounces
Egg	1	Potato	1 serving	Potato	1 serving
Cereal*	1 serving	Vegetable	1 serving	Vegetable	1 serving
Toast*	1 slice	Salad	1 serving	Salad	1 serving
Fat	3 teaspoons	Bread*	1 slice	Bread*	1 slice
Sugar, jelly	2 tablespoons	Fat	3 teaspoons	Fat	3 teaspoons
Beverage	1 cup	Fruit	1 serving	Milk	1 cup
		Milk	1 cup	Dessert*	1 serving
		Sugar, jelly	1 tablespoon	Sugar, jelly	1 tablespoon
		Beverage	1 cup	Beverage	1 cup

*Note limitations listed on page 54.

FOOD GROUPS

Allowed	Omitted
Beverage	
Coffee, tea, decaffeinated coffee; carbonated beverage	Cereal beverage; prepared drinks with malt, wheat, rye, oats, or barley*
Meat	
Meat, fish, fowl; egg; cottage cheese, cheese except "Omitted"; peanut butter	Any prepared with wheat, rye, oats, or barley; processed meats or cheese*
Fat	
Any except "Omitted"	Commercial salad dressings*
Milk	
Any except "Omitted"	Commercial chocolate milk*; prepared milk drinks made with cereal additive or malt
Bread	
Bread made with wheat starch, arrowroot, corn, potato, rice, or soybean flour; gluten-free bread mix	Any made with wheat (except wheat starch), rye, oats, barley, or buckwheat
Corn or rice cereals (malt flavoring allowed as tolerated)	Any other
Potato and potato substitutes except "Omitted"	Macaroni, noodles, spaghetti; any prepared with wheat (except wheat starch), rye, oats, buckwheat, or barley
Vegetable	
Any prepared with "Allowed" foods	
Fruit	
Any prepared with "Allowed" foods	
Soup	
Broth, bouillon, or vegetable soup; cream soups thickened with "Allowed" flours or starches	Soups made with wheat, rye, oats, or barley; commercial soups
Dessert	
Gelatin; cake, cookies, pastries, puddings prepared with allowed flours or starches; sherbet, ice cream*	Any made with wheat, rye, oats, or barley; commercially prepared mixes

Allowed	Omitted

Sweets

Any except "Omitted"

Commercial candy with wheat, rye, oats, or barley*

Miscellaneous

Salt, spices, herbs; vinegar; pickles; sauces and gravies prepared with flours or starches "Allowed"; baking chocolate, cocoa powder *

Bottled meat sauces, pickles or condiments with wheat, rye, oats, or barley; flavoring syrups,* cocoa mixes*

*Consult list of contents on label or check with the manufacturer.

FAT-RESTRICTED DIET FOR STEATORRHEA (OTHER THAN GLUTEN-INDUCED SPRUE)

70 Gram Fat, 50 Gram Fat, and 30 Gram Fat Diets

APPROXIMATE COMPOSITION (10 to 15% Variation)

Diet	Protein	Fat	Carbohydrate	Calories	Sodium*	Potassium	Fluid
	gm	gm	gm		mEq	mEq	ml
70 Gram Fat	115	70	335	2,430	140	120	2,500
50 Gram Fat	90	50	355	2,230	125	105	2,500
30 Gram Fat	80	30	365	2,050	100	100	2,500

*Value is for average amount of salt used in preparation of food; salt added to food at the table is not calculated.

GENERAL INFORMATION

The fat-restricted diets may be used in the management of patients with steatorrhea due to disorders other than gluten sensitivity. The diets are moderately restricted in fiber. The physician should *specify* the level of fat desired. If medium chain triglycerides are to be included in the dietary regimen, the physician should indicate the desired amount. See page 141 for discussion of medium chain triglycerides.

Diets available are as follows:

70 Gram Fat. The diet provides 65% or more protein than is suggested for adults. Approximately 24% of the total calories are derived from fat.

50 Gram Fat. The diet may be ordered if the 70 Gram Fat Diet is not tolerated. It provides 30% or more protein than is suggested for adults. Approximately 20% of the total calories come from fat.

30 Gram Fat. The diet meets the protein requirements of adults. The level of protein may be increased by supplementing the diet with powdered skim milk. Fat and oils are eliminated unless the physician has ordered medium chain triglycerides to be included in the diet. Less than 15% of the total calories come from fat.

The diets are planned with the Mayo Clinic Food Exchange List. Servings of food exchanges are suggested in the following table. This table should be used only as a guide in planning the diets. Modifications within the prescribed dietary restrictions may be made in order to adapt the diet to the normal dietary pattern of the hospital or the patient.

SUGGESTED DAILY FOOD EXCHANGES (Mayo Clinic Food Exchange List, inside covers)

Diet	Meat	Skim milk*	Fat†	Bread	Vegetable*	Fruit*	Dessert*	Sweets*
70 Gram Fat	10	3	3	9	3–4	5–6	1	4
50 Gram Fat	6	3	3	9	3–4	5–6	1	5
30 Gram Fat	5	3‡	...	7	3–4	6–7	1	6

*Amount not restricted.
†Medium chain triglycerides may be used in addition to dietary fat.
‡Diets may be supplemented with powdered skim milk if a higher protein level is desired.

SUGGESTED MENU PATTERNS

	70 Gram Fat Diet	50 Gram Fat Diet	30 Gram Fat Diet
Breakfast			
Fruit	2 servings	2 servings	2 servings
Cereal	1 serving	1 serving	1 serving
Egg	1	1	1
Toast	2 slices	2 slices	1 slice
Fat	1 teaspoon	1 teaspoon	...
Skim milk	1 cup	1 cup	1 cup
Sugar, jelly	2 tablespoons	2 tablespoons	2 tablespoons
Beverage	1 cup	1 cup	1 cup
Noon Meal			
Meat	4 ounces	2 ounces	2 ounces
Potato	1 serving	1 serving	1 serving
Vegetable	1 serving	1 serving	1 serving
Salad	1 serving	1 serving	1 serving
Bread	2 slices	2 slices	1 slice
Fat	1 teaspoon	1 teaspoon	...
Fruit	2 servings	2 servings	2 servings
Skim milk	1 cup	1 cup	1 cup
Sugar, jelly	1 tablespoon	1 tablespoon	2 tablespoons
Beverage	1 cup	1 cup	1 cup
Evening Meal			
Meat	5 ounces	3 ounces	2 ounces
Potato	1 serving	1 serving	1 serving
Vegetable	1 serving	1 serving	1 serving
Salad	1 serving	1 serving	1 serving
Bread	2 slices	2 slices	2 slices
Fat	1 teaspoon	1 teaspoon	...
Dessert	1 serving	1 serving	1 serving
Skim milk	1 cup	1 cup	1 cup
Sugar, jelly	1 tablespoon	2 tablespoons	2 tablespoons
Beverage	1 cup	1 cup	1 cup

FOOD GROUPS

Allowed	Omitted
	Fried foods
Beverage	
Coffee, tea; cereal beverage; carbonated beverage	
Meat	
Meat, fish, or fowl without visible fat or skin; egg; cottage cheese	Fried; fish canned in oil; other cheese; peanut butter
Fat	
Any except "Omitted"	Avocado; olives; nuts
Milk	
Skim milk, buttermilk (fat free), powdered skim milk	Any other
Bread	
Refined wheat, rye, or graham bread, rolls, or crackers	Any with whole grain flour, bran, seeds, nuts, butter, or cheese; quick breads
Refined cereals–cooked or ready to eat	Whole grain or bran cereal
Potato and potato substitutes; puréed corn, lima beans, peas; hominy grits	Whole grain rice; dried legumes; popcorn; potato chips, fried potatoes
Vegetable	
Canned or cooked mild-flavored vegetables or juice without seeds or coarse fiber; lettuce, tomato (no seeds or skin)	Any other raw; strong flavored
Fruit	
Canned or cooked fruit without seeds or skin; fruit juice; banana, citrus fruits without membrane	Any other
Soup	
Fat free broth, bouillon or any made with "Allowed" vegetables and milk	Commercial soups; any made with whole milk or cream
Dessert	
Angel food or sponge cake, low fat cookies; gelatin, pudding; sherbet	Any with butter, chocolate, coconut, cream, nuts, whole milk, or "Omitted" fruits; commercially prepared mixes
Sweets	
Any except "Omitted"	Jam, marmalade; candy with chocolate, cream, fat, coconut, nuts, or "Omitted" fruits
Miscellaneous	
Salt; spices and herbs except "Omitted"; condiments; vinegar; cocoa	Garlic, seed spices; pickles; gravy, white sauce; chocolate

LACTOSE INTOLERANCE

Lactose-Restricted Diet

NUTRITIONAL ADEQUACY

This diet is low in calcium; it is adequate in all other nutrients according to the Recommended Daily Dietary Allowances of the National Research Council.

APPROXIMATE COMPOSITION (10 to 15% Variation)

Protein	Fat	Carbohydrate	Calories	Calcium	Sodium*	Potassium	Fluid
gm	gm	gm		gm	mEq	mEq	ml
70	90	235	2,030	0.16	125	75	1,700

*Value is for average amount of salt used in preparation of food; salt added to food at the table is not calculated.

GENERAL INFORMATION

The Lactose-Restricted Diet is designed to provide a minimal amount of lactose (8 gm or less) per day. Labels of food products should be checked for addition of milk, lactose, and milk solids. When these are listed as major ingredients, the food should be avoided or used as tolerated. Lactate, lactalbumin, and calcium compounds are salts of lactic acid and do not contain lactose.

The Lactose-Restricted Diet is planned with the Mayo Clinic Food Exchange List. Servings of food exchanges are suggested in the following table. This table should be used only as a guide in planning the diet. Modifications within the prescribed dietary restrictions may be made in order to adapt the diet to the normal dietary pattern of the hospital or the patient.

SUGGESTED DAILY FOOD EXCHANGES* (Mayo Clinic Food Exchange List, inside covers)

Meat	Fat	Milk	Bread	Vegetable	Fruit	Dessert	Sweets
7	11	...	8	3–4	2–3	1	4

*Amounts not restricted.

SUGGESTED MENU PATTERN

Breakfast		Noon Meal		Evening Meal	
Fruit	1 serving	Meat	3 ounces	Meat	3 ounces
Egg	1	Potato	1 serving	Potato	1 serving
Cereal	1 serving	Vegetable	1 serving	Vegetable	1 serving
Toast	1 slice	Salad	1 serving	Salad	1 serving
Fat	5 teaspoons	Bread	2 slices	Bread	2 slices
Sugar, jelly	2 tablespoons	Fat	3 teaspoons	Fat	3 teaspoons
Beverage	1 cup	Fruit	1 serving	Dessert	1 serving
		Sugar, jelly	1 tablespoon	Sugar, jelly	1 tablespoon
		Beverage	1 cup	Beverage	1 cup

FOOD GROUPS

Allowed	Omitted
Foods processed with minor amounts of milk, milk solids, or lactose may be used with discretion, if tolerated	

Beverage

Allowed	Omitted
Coffee, tea; carbonated beverage; cereal beverage	Prepared drinks with milk or milk products*

Meat

Allowed	Omitted
Meat, fish, or fowl; egg; peanut butter	Any prepared or processed with milk or milk products*; cottage cheese, cheese

Fat

Allowed	Omitted
Any except "Omitted"; nondairy cream substitutes*; half and half(1/3 cup or less per day)	Margarine and salad dressings with added milk or milk products; cream cheese, sour cream, whipped cream

Milk

Allowed	Omitted
1/3 cup or less may be used in place of cream allowance	Any milk or milk products except "Allowed"

Bread

Allowed	Omitted
Bread, quick breads, rolls, crackers, cereals except "Omitted"	Any prepared or processed with milk products; commercially prepared mixes; certain dry cereals*
Potato and potato substitutes; dried legumes; popcorn	Any creamed

Vegetable

Allowed	Omitted
Any except "Omitted"	Vegetables processed or prepared with milk or milk products

Fruit

Allowed	Omitted
Any	

Soup

Allowed	Omitted
Bouillon, broth, or soups made of "Allowed" foods	Cream soups; commercial soups with milk or milk products

Dessert

Allowed	Omitted
Fruit ice; gelatin; cake, cookies, pastries made without milk or milk products	Any with milk or milk products: sherbet, ice cream, pudding; commercial desserts or mixes*

Allowed	Omitted

Sweets

Any except "Omitted"; pure sugar candy	Cream or chocolate candies; commercial candy containing milk or milk products; molasses

Miscellaneous

Salt, spices, herbs; condiments; gravy; pickles; vinegar	White sauce, milk chocolate, cocoa mixes*

*Consult list of contents on label or check with the manufacturer.

GOUT

PURINE-FREE DIET, LOW PURINE DIET

APPROXIMATE COMPOSITION (10 to 15% Variation)

Diet	Protein	Fat	Carbohydrate	Calories	Sodium*	Potassium	Fluid
	gm	gm	gm		mEq	mEq	ml
Purine-free	70	95	230	2,055	115	70	1,800
Low Purine	70	95	230	2,055	110	80	2,000

*Value is for average amount of salt used in preparation of food; salt which may be added to food at the table is not calculated.

GENERAL INFORMATION

A purine-restricted diet may be ordered as a supplement to drug therapy in the management of increased levels of blood uric acid. Diets with two levels of purine are available. The level of fat in the diets should not exceed 40% of the calories.

Purine-Free Diet. This diet may be used during acute characteristic symptoms. Foods with high or moderate purine content are omitted. (See next table, groups 2 and 3.) Egg (one per day), peanut butter, cheese, and other dairy products are substituted for meat, fish, or fowl. Foods in group 1 may be used as desired.

Low Purine Diet. This diet may be used during remission of symptoms of gout. Foods with high purine content are omitted (group 3); foods with moderate purine content may be used daily in prescribed amounts (group 2). Foods in group 1 may be used as desired.

Purine Content of Foods

Group 1: negligible, 0–15 mg	Group 2: moderate, 50–150 mg	Group 3: high, 150–800 mg
Cheese	Meats	Wild game
Egg	Fish, shellfish	Organ meats
Milk	Fowl	Goose
Bread	Dried legumes	Anchovies, herring, sardines, mackerel, scallops
Cereal	Asparagus	
Fruit	Spinach	Broth, meat extracts
Vegetable (except group 2)	Peas	Gravy
Sugar		

The purine-restricted diets are planned with the Mayo Clinic Food Exchange List. The meat group has been divided into two groups: meat and meat substitutes.

Servings of food exchanges for each diet are suggested in the following table. This table should be used only as a guide in planning the diets. Modifications within the prescribed dietary restrictions may be made in order to adapt the diet to the normal dietary pattern of the hospital or the patient.

SUGGESTED DAILY FOOD EXCHANGES (Mayo Clinic Food Exchange
List, inside covers)

Diet	Meat	Meat substitute*	Fat	Milk	Bread[†]	Vegetable[†]	Fruit[†]	Dessert[†]	Sweets[†]
Purine-Free	...	5	9	2	6	3–4	2–3	1	4
Low Purine	4	1	9	2	6	3–4	2–3	1	4

*Meat substitutes: egg (one per day), peanut butter, cottage cheese, cheese, other dairy products.
†Amount not restricted.

SUGGESTED MENU PATTERN

	Purine-Free Diet	Low Purine Diet
Breakfast		
Fruit	1 serving	1 serving
Egg	1	1
Cereal	1 serving	1 serving
Toast	1 slice	1 slice
Fat	3 teaspoons	3 teaspoons
Sugar, jelly	2 tablespoons	2 tablespoons
Beverage	1 cup	1 cup
Noon Meal		
Meat or substitute	2*	2 ounces
Potato	1 serving	1 serving
Vegetable	1 serving	1 serving
Salad	1 serving	1 serving
Bread	1 slice	1 slice
Fat	3 teaspoons	3 teaspoons
Fruit	1 serving	1 serving
Milk	1 cup	1 cup
Sugar, jelly	1 tablespoon	1 tablespoon
Beverage	1 cup	1 cup
Evening Meal		
Meat or substitute	2*	2 ounces
Potato	1 serving	1 serving
Vegetable	1 serving	1 serving
Salad	1 serving	1 serving
Bread	1 slice	1 slice
Fat	3 teaspoons	3 teaspoons
Dessert	1 serving	1 serving
Milk	1 cup	1 cup
Sugar, jelly	1 tablespoon	1 tablespoon
Beverage	1 cup	1 cup

*Meat substitutes: peanut butter, cheese, cottage cheese, or other dairy products.

FOOD GROUPS

Allowed	Omitted
	Fried foods
Beverage	
Coffee, tea; carbonated beverage; cereal beverage	
Meat	
Meat, fish, or fowl (group 2) ; egg; cheese; peanut butter	Fried; wild game; goose; anchovies, herring, mackerel, sardines; scallops; heart, kidney, liver, sweetbreads (group 3)
Meat substitutes	
Egg; peanut butter; cottage cheese, cheese, other dairy products	
Fat	
Any except "Omitted"	Bacon
Milk	
Milk, milk drinks	
Bread	
Any except "Omitted"; dried legumes and peas may be used with discretion	Fried potato, potato chips
Vegetable	
Any; vegetables in group 2 may be used with discretion	
Fruit	
Any	
Soup	
Any except "Omitted"	Broth, bouillon; commercial soups
Dessert	
Any	
Sweets	
Any	
Miscellaneous	
Salt, spices, herbs; condiments, pickles; vinegar; white sauce; chocolate, cocoa	Gravy

DISEASES OF THE LIVER

30 GRAM PROTEIN AND 120 GRAM PROTEIN DIETS

NUTRITIONAL ADEQUACY

The 30 Gram Protein Diet is inadequate in B vitamins and minerals.

The 120 Gram Protein Diet is nutritionally adequate according to the Recommended Daily Dietary Allowances of the National Research Council.

APPROXIMATE COMPOSITION (10 to 15% Variation)

Diet	Protein gm	Fat gm	Carbohydrate gm	Calories	Sodium* mEq	Potassium mEq	Fluid ml
30 Gram Protein	30	90	335	2,270	60	45	1,600
120 Gram Protein	120	145	315	3,000	160	115	2,500

*Value is for average amount of salt used in preparation of food; salt added to food at the table is not calculated.

GENERAL INFORMATION

In the management of liver disease, diets with modifications in protein content may be indicated as part of the treatment. The physician should order a diet in accordance with the severity of the patient's condition.

30 Gram Protein Diet.   In severe disorders of the liver, the 30 Gram Protein Diet may be ordered. Sources of protein from fruits and vegetables are calculated in this diet: one serving of fruit contains 0.5 gm of protein; one serving of vegetable contains 1 gm protein.

120 Gram Protein Diet.   In mild disorders of the liver, the 120 Gram Protein Diet may be ordered. Additional calories may be provided by an increase in carbohydrates and protein. A moderate amount of fat may be included to make the diet palatable. If necessary, the physician may order a diet containing more than 120 gm of protein.

Diets with moderate protein content may be ordered by the physician. Daily food allowances for diets between 30 and 120 gm of protein are suggested in the section "Renal Diseases," page 77.

Dietary patterns are not given for diets with less than 30 gm of protein. Individualization of these diets will be necessary.

Protein Content of Food Groups.   Each food group, as outlined on pages 69 and 70, contains foods similar to those of food groups in the Mayo Clinic Food Exchange List. One exception is made in the "Fat" group (page 69). Because of their protein content, cream and other dairy products usually listed in the "Fat" group are listed in a separate category, "Milk Products." Various forms of milk and frozen dairy desserts also are listed under this category. The amount of each food that can be used in place of 1/2 cup of milk is specified.

An additional category, "Low Protein Bread Products," is included. The foods in this group are to be made from wheat starch, cornstarch, tapioca, arrowroot, or low protein bread mix. Because the table gives the composition for bread only, nutrient values for other products made with low protein flours should be calculated individually. Other foods that contribute negligible amounts of protein are given in a table on page 80.

The 30 Gram Protein Diet and the 120 Gram Protein Diet are planned with the Mayo Clinic Food Exchange List. The dietary program for the 30 Gram Protein Diet should also include the food groups given in the two foregoing paragraphs. Servings of food exchanges are suggested for each diet in the following table. This table should be used only as a guide in planning the diets. Modifications within the prescribed dietary restrictions may be made in order to adapt the diet to the normal dietary pattern of the hospital or the patient.

SUGGESTED DAILY FOOD EXCHANGES (Mayo Clinic Food Exchange List, inside covers)

Diet	Meat	Fat	Milk	Bread	Low protein products	Vegetable	Fruit	Dessert	Sweets
30 Gram Protein	3	10*	1/2	1	5†	2	6	...	4*
120 Gram Protein*	10	9	3	9	...	3–4	2–3	2	4

*Foods not restricted.

†Low protein bread and desserts should be prepared from wheat starch, cornstarch, arrowroot, tapioca, or low protein bread mix.

Sodium Restrictions.   Diets with sodium and protein restrictions may be ordered by the physician. Appropriate diets to use are found in the section on "Renal Diseases," page 77.

SUGGESTED MENU PATTERN

	30 Gram Protein Diet	120 Gram Protein Diet
Breakfast		
Fruit	2 servings	1 serving
Egg	1	1
Cereal	1 serving	1 serving
Toast	1 slice*	2 slices
Fat	2 teaspoons	3 teaspoons
Milk	1/2 cup	1 cup
Sugar, jelly	2 tablespoons	2 tablespoons
Beverage	1 cup	1 cup
Noon Meal		
Meat	1 ounce	4 ounces
Potato	...	1 serving
Vegetable	1 serving	1 serving
Salad	...	1 serving
Bread	2 slices*	2 slices
Fat	3 teaspoons	3 teaspoons
Fruit	2 servings	1 serving
Dessert	...	1 serving
Milk	...	1 cup
Sugar, jelly	1 tablespoon	1 tablespoon
Beverage	1 cup	1 cup
Evening Meal		
Meat	1 ounce	5 ounces
Potato	...	1 serving
Vegetable	1 serving	1 serving
Salad	1 serving	1 serving
Bread	2 slices*	2 slices
Fat	4 teaspoons	3 teaspoons
Dessert	2 servings (fruit)	1 serving
Milk	...	1 cup
Sugar, jelly	1 tablespoon	1 tablespoon
Beverage	1 cup	1 cup

*Low protein bread or bread products.

FOOD GROUPS

30 Gram Protein Diet

Allowed	*Omitted*

Beverage
Coffee, tea; carbonated beverage; cereal beverage

Meat
Meat, fish, fowl; egg; cheese; peanut butter

Fat

Butter, margarine, cooking fats; salad dressings	Bacon; nuts

Milk

1/2 cup of milk per day	Any in excess of "Allowed"

Milk Products
The following may be used in place of 1/2 cup
   of milk:

Milk

Condensed	1/4 cup
Dry	2 tablespoons
Evaporated	1/4 cup
Yogurt	1/2 cup

Cream

Half and half	1/2 cup
Sour	1/2 cup
Whipped	2/3 cup
Cream cheese	4 tablespoons

Frozen Desserts

Ice cream	1/2 cup
Ice milk	1/3 cup
Sherbet	1 cup

Bread

Only **one** serving of **one** of the following per day: bread, cereal, potato, or potato substitute	Cereal with protein concentrates; dried legumes; corn, lima beans, peas; popcorn

Low Protein Bread Products

Bread, rolls, quick breads, or desserts made with wheat starch, cornstarch, arrowroot, tapioca, or low protein baking mix	Any prepared with egg, milk, or milk products unless part of "Allowed" food

Vegetable
Any

Fruit
Any

Allowed	*Omitted*

Soup

Any made with "Allowed" foods

Dessert

Fruit ice; see "Milk Products" and "Low Pro-   Any other
tein Bread Products" for additional desserts

Sweets

Any except "Omitted"   Chocolate, cream, or filled candy or any made
with foods not "Allowed"

Miscellaneous

Salt, spices, herbs; condiments; flavoring ex-   Milk chocolate, instant cocoa mixes
tracts; baking chocolate, cocoa powder;
pickles, vinegar; gravy and white sauce
made with "Allowed" milk

120 Gram Protein Diet

All foods are allowed. Emphasis should be placed on protein and carbohydrate foods as sources of calories.

OBESITY

CALORIE-RESTRICTED DIETS

800 Calorie, 1,000 Calorie, 1,200 Calorie, and 1,400 Calorie Diets

NUTRITIONAL ADEQUACY

The Calorie-Restricted Diets of 1,000 calories or more are nutritionally adequate according to the Recommended Daily Dietary Allowances of the National Research Council. The physician may wish to prescribe vitamin and mineral supplements for diets of less than 1,000 calories.

APPROXIMATE COMPOSITION (10 to 15% Variation)

Diet	Protein gm	Fat gm	Carbohydrate gm	Sodium* mEq	Potassium mEq	Fluid ml
800 Calorie	60	30	80	55	70	1,800
1,000 Calorie	70	40	90	65	75	1,800
1,200 Calorie	75	50	120	85	85	1,900
1,400 Calorie	75	70	120	85	85	1,900

*Value is for average amount of salt used in preparation of food; salt which may be added to food at the table is not calculated.

GENERAL INFORMATION

Calorie-Restricted Diets may be ordered as "weighed" or "not weighed." A Prediction-of-Weight-Loss Chart will be calculated routinely for all patients instructed in a Weighed 800 Calorie Diet or for any patient indicated by the physician. Patients are asked to return their weight-loss charts by mail to their physician at 9-week intervals. The dietitian will send a revised Prediction-of-Weight-Loss Chart to the patient. See Method of Predicting Weight Loss (page 72).

The Calorie-Restricted Diets are planned according to the Mayo Clinic Food Exchange List. Servings of food exchanges for each diet are suggested in the following table. This table should be used only as a guide in planning the diets. Modifications within the prescribed dietary restriction may be made in order to adapt the diet to the normal dietary pattern of the hospital or the patient.

SUGGESTED DAILY FOOD EXCHANGES (Mayo Clinic Food Exchange List, inside covers)

Diet	Meat	Milk	Fat	Bread	Vegetable	Fruit
800 Calorie	6	2*	...	1	3–4	3
1,000 Calorie	7	2*	1	2	3–4	3
1,200 Calorie	7	2*	3	4	3–4	3
1,400 Calorie	7	2	3	4	3–4	3

*Skim milk or buttermilk (fat free).

Method of Predicting Loss of Weight[1]

Determine the individual's basal caloric requirement for 24 hours according to the directions on the food nomogram (page 160). Weigh and measure the patient without shoes.

The weight to be used in the determination of the basal caloric requirement is 15 pounds less than the actual weight. If the actual weight does not exceed the ideal weight by 15 pounds or more, it is preferable to use the ideal weight for this determination. To the basal caloric requirement for adults, add an increase of 10 to 40% (usually 20%) for activity.

For children 5 to 10 years of age, add an increase of 70% to the basal caloric requirement for activity, and for anyone 10 to 20 years of age add 50%. In all cases, the increase added to the basal caloric requirement depends on the degree of activity of the individual. It should be increased for persons who are more active than average and decreased for those who are less active.

The resulting figure is an estimate of the average daily expenditure of energy expressed in calories.

The difference between the calories expended and the calories consumed is termed the "calorie deficit." This figure multiplied by the factor 0.002[2] will give the estimated loss of weight per week in pounds. A graph can be constructed to show the predicted loss of weight from day to day.

EXAMPLE OF PREDICTION OF LOSS OF WEIGHT

Female: age, 36 years   **Actual weight:** 230 pounds
Height: 5 feet 3 inches   **Ideal weight:** 125 pounds

230 pounds − 15 pounds = 215 pounds

Basal calories for 215 pounds from the food nomogram = 1,700

Basal calories plus 20% of basal calories = 2,040 calories

Calorie deficit: 2,040 calories − 800 calories (provided in diet) = 1,240 calories

Estimated loss of weight per week: 1,240 calories × 0.002 = 2.5 pounds (see graph, page 73)

The rate of loss of weight is recalculated at the end of every 9 weeks.

---

[1]Gastineau, C. F.: The prediction of weight loss on a reducing diet. (Editorial) Minn. Med. *43:* 255–257 (Apr.) 1960.

[2]The factor 0.002 is obtained as follows: D (calorie deficit) ÷ 9.3 = grams of fat lost per day. Grams of fat lost per day $\times \frac{100}{86}$ = grams of weight lost per day, when fat tissue contains 14% of water. Grams of weight lost per day × 7 = grams of weight lost per week. Grams of weight lost per week $\times \frac{2.2}{1,000}$ = pounds lost per week. Thus, the pounds lost per week $= \frac{D}{9.3} \times \frac{100}{86} \times 7 \times \frac{2.2}{1,000} = D \times 0.00193$ or approximately $D \times 0.002$.

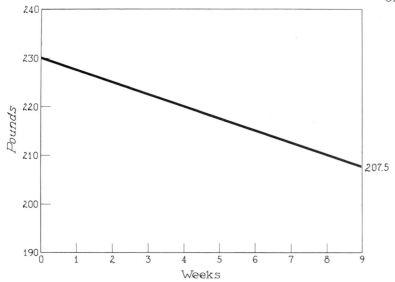

SUGGESTED MENU PATTERN

	800 Calorie Diet	1,000 Calorie Diet	1,200 Calorie Diet	1,400 Calorie Diet
Breakfast				
Fruit	1 serving	1 serving	1 serving	1 serving
Egg	1	1	1	1
Toast	1 slice	1 slice	1 slice	1 slice
Fat	...	1 teaspoon	1 teaspoon	1 teaspoon
Beverage	1 cup	1 cup	1 cup	1 cup
Noon Meal				
Meat	2 ounces	3 ounces	3 ounces	3 ounces
Vegetable	1 serving	1 serving	1 serving	1 serving
Salad	1 serving	1 serving	1 serving	1 serving
Bread	...	...	1 slice	1 slice
Fat	...	...	1 teaspoon	1 teaspoon
Fruit	1 serving	1 serving	1 serving	1 serving
Milk	1 cup*	1 cup*	1 cup*	1 cup
Beverage	1 cup	1 cup	1 cup	1 cup
Evening Meal				
Meat	3 ounces	3 ounces	3 ounces	3 ounces
Potato	...	1 serving	1 serving	1 serving
Vegetable	1 serving	1 serving	1 serving	1 serving
Salad	1 serving	1 serving	1 serving	1 serving
Bread	...	...	1 slice	1 slice
Fat	...	...	1 teaspoon	1 teaspoon
Fruit	1 serving	1 serving	1 serving	1 serving
Milk	1 cup*	1 cup*	1 cup*	1 cup
Beverage	1 cup	1 cup	1 cup	1 cup

*Skim milk or buttermilk (fat free).

MAINTENANCE OF WEIGHT DURING PREGNANCY

1,200 CALORIE REDUCTION DIET
AND
1,800 CALORIE WEIGHT MAINTENANCE DIET

NUTRITIONAL ADEQUACY

The physician may wish to order vitamin and mineral supplements when considered necessary.

APPROXIMATE COMPOSITION (10 to 15% Variation)

Diet	Protein gm	Fat gm	Carbohydrate gm	Sodium* mEq	Potassium mEq	Fluid ml
1,200 Calorie Reduction	85	50	105	70	95	2,300
1,800 Calorie Weight Maintenance†	100	70	190	105	115	2,400

*Value is for a moderate amount of salt used in preparation of food; salt is not to be added at the table.
†Calories may be adjusted to meet individual needs for weight maintenance.

GENERAL INFORMATION

Control of weight is desired during pregnancy in order to avoid possible complications and discomfort. Weight gained during the last 6 months of pregnancy should not exceed $2\frac{1}{2}$ pounds per month.

1,200 Calorie Reduction Diet.   The diet may be ordered for a woman who exceeds the recommended weight gain or who is overweight prior to pregnancy. The diet also may be used as a weight maintenance regimen for those who require fewer calories to maintain a desirable weight.

1,800 Calorie Weight Maintenance Diet.   The diet may be ordered for a woman who requires 1,800 calories to maintain a desirable weight. Although the Recommended Daily Dietary Allowances of the National Research Council indicates a caloric intake of more than 1,800 calories during pregnancy, calories should be adjusted to meet individual needs for weight maintenance.

The diets to be used during pregnancy may include foods prepared or processed with salt. Additional salt should not be used at mealtime.

The diets recommended for maintenance of desirable weight during pregnancy are planned with the Mayo Clinic Food Exchange List. Food exchanges are suggested for each diet in the following table. The table should be used only as a guide in planning the diets. Modifications within the prescribed dietary restrictions may be made in order to adapt the diet to the normal dietary pattern of the hospital or the patient.

SUGGESTED DAILY FOOD EXCHANGES (Mayo Clinic Food Exchange List, inside covers)

Diet	Meat	Fat	Skim milk	Bread	Vegetable	Fruit	Dessert	Sweets
1,200 Calorie Reduction	7*	3	4	1	4	3†	...	...
1,800 Calorie Weight Maintenance	8*	4	4	4	4	3†	1	...

*A serving of liver should be included each week.
†A serving of citrus fruit or other foods high in vitamin C should be included each day.

Dry Diet. Dry, solid foods may be ordered if nausea and vomiting occur. Six small meals should be served without liquids or foods of fluid consistency. Liquids are allowed 1 hour before and after meals. When nausea and vomiting subside, other foods are added as tolerated.

Diet During Lactation. The diet during lactation should be reasonably high in calories. The caloric level of the diet should be adjusted for weight maintenance.

SUGGESTED MENU PATTERN

	1,200 Calorie Reduction Diet	1,800 Calorie Weight Maintenance Diet
Breakfast		
Fruit	1 serving*	1 serving
Egg	1	1
Toast	1 slice	1 slice
Fat	1 teaspoon	1 teaspoon
Beverage	1 cup	1 cup
Noon Meal		
Meat	3 ounces	3 ounces
Vegetable	1 serving	1 serving
Salad	1 serving	1 serving
Bread	...	1 slice
Fat	1 teaspoon	1 teaspoon
Fruit	1 serving*	1 serving
Milk, skim	1 cup	1 cup
Beverage	1 cup	1 cup
Evening Meal		
Meat	3 ounces	4 ounces
Potato	...	1 serving
Vegetable	1 serving	1 serving
Salad	1 serving	1 serving
Bread	...	1 slice
Fat	1 teaspoon	2 teaspoons
Dessert	1 serving*	1 serving
Milk, skim	1 cup	1 cup
Beverage	1 cup	1 cup
Between-Meal Feedings (3 and 8 p. m.)		
Milk, skim	1 cup	1 cup
Fruit	...	1 serving

*Unsweetened fruit.

RENAL DISEASES

CONTROLLED PROTEIN, SODIUM, AND POTASSIUM DIETS FOR ADULTS

NUTRITIONAL ADEQUACY

The 30 Gram Protein Diets are inadequate in calcium and folic acid and low in phosphorus, thiamine, niacin, and riboflavin. The 50 Gram Protein Diets are inadequate in calcium and low in phosphorus, thiamine, riboflavin, niacin, and folic acid. The 70, the 100, and the 120 gram protein diets are nutritionally adequate according to the Recommended Daily Dietary Allowances of the National Research Council.

APPROXIMATE COMPOSITION (10 to 15% Variation)

Diet	Protein gm	Fat gm	Carbohydrate gm	Calories*	Sodium mEq	Potassium mEq	Fluid ml
30 Gram Protein (20, 40, 90 mEq sodium)	30	85	410	2,500	20, 40, or 90†	45	1,500
50 Gram Protein (20, 40, 90 mEq sodium)	50	85	405	2,550	20, 40, or 90†	65	1,800
70 Gram Protein (20, 40, 90 mEq sodium)	70	85	390	2,600	20, 40, or 90†	85	2,200
100 Gram Protein (30, 40, 90 mEq sodium)	100	105	315	2,600	30, 40, or 90†	95	2,200
120 Gram Protein (90 mEq sodium)	120	125	245	2,600	90	95	2,300

*Calories may be modified by the addition or restriction of foods from Carbohydrate (CHO) Supplement Group, page 86.
†The physician should specify desired level of sodium when ordering a diet.

GENERAL INFORMATION

Sodium Restrictions.   The 30, 50, and 70 gram protein diets for renal diseases may be planned with 20, 40, or 90 mEq of sodium. Because of the natural sodium content of protein foods, the 100 Gram Protein Diet is planned with minimal sodium (30 mEq) and the 120 Gram Protein Diet is planned with 90 mEq of sodium. The use of dialyzed or low sodium milk or the reduction of the amount of regular milk may be necessary if a severer restriction is ordered.

Potassium Restrictions.   The diets for renal diseases are planned with 100 mEq or less of potassium. If necessary, the physician may order a diet with a specific level of potassium. Fruits and vegetables are divided into two groups (1 and 2) according to the content of potassium. Diets ordered without a specific level of potassium restrictions may include foods from both groups.

Fluid Content of Diets.   The water content of foods is included in the fluid values listed for each diet. The physician may order a specific level of fluids if necessary.

Patients being instructed on diets of 20 mEq of sodium or less are advised to check the sodium level of their local water supply. If the sodium level exceeds 40 parts per million (2 mEq per quart), distilled water should be used. Chemically softened water should not be used on any sodium-restricted diet.

Diets With Less Than 30 Grams of Protein.   Diet plans are not given for protein levels of less than 30 gm because research concerning severely restricted protein diets is presently in progress. These diets should be individualized according to the physician's order for the patient. Consideration should be given to current research which may indicate the most beneficial form of diet therapy.

MODIFIED MAYO CLINIC FOOD EXCHANGE LISTS

The food exchange list used in planning diets for renal diseases is based on protein, sodium, and potassium content of foods. Modifications of the Mayo Clinic Food Exchange List were made (pages 81 to 86). Average values for each food group are given in the table on page 80. This table may be used for a quick calculation of dietary composition. When more accurate figures are desired, the table on Sodium and Potassium Content of Foods in Mayo Clinic Food Exchange List Appendix, pages 143 to 147 should be consulted.

SUGGESTED SERVINGS OF FOOD EXCHANGES

Servings of food exchanges from the Mayo Clinic Food Exchange List for Controlled Protein, Sodium, and Potassium Diets are suggested in the table on page 79. This table should be used only as a guide in planning a diet. Modifications within the prescribed dietary restrictions may be made in order to adapt the diet to the normal dietary meal pattern of the hospital or the patient.

Attention must be given to providing minimal daily requirements of essential amino acids in order to maintain nitrogen balance and to providing sufficient calories to maintain body weight.

SUGGESTED MENU PATTERN

Food exchanges for the **30 Gram Protein, 20 mEq Sodium Diet (less than 100 mEq potassium)** may be served as suggested below.

Breakfast		Noon Meal		Evening Meal	
Fruit	1 serving	Meat	1 ounce	Meat	1 ounce
Egg	1	Vegetable*	1 serving	Vegetable	1 serving
Cereal	1 serving	Bread, low protein	2 slices	Bread, low protein	2 slices
Bread, low protein	2 slices	Fat	4 teaspoons	Fat	4 teaspoons
Fat	3 teaspoons	Fruit	1 serving	Fruit	2 servings
Milk products	1/2 cup	CHO supplement	2 servings	CHO supplement	2 servings
CHO supplement	2 servings	Beverage	1 cup	Beverage	1 cup
Beverage	1 cup				

*Salted in preparation or processing.

SUGGESTED DAILY FOOD EXCHANGES (see pages 81 to 86 for size of portions)

Diet	Meat	Fat	Milk or milk products*	Bread	Low protein bread	Vege- table	Fruit	Carbo- hydrate supple- ment	Bever- age	Salt (sha- ker)†
30 Gram Protein: 45 mEq										
potassium, 1,500 ml fluid										
20 mEq Na	3	11	1	1	6	2†	4	6	3	...
40 mEq Na	3	11	1	1	6	2†	4	6	3	1/4 tsp
90 mEq Na	3†	11†	1	1†	6	2†	4	6	3	1/4 tsp
50 Gram Protein: 65 mEq										
potassium, 1,800 ml fluid										
20 mEq Na	5(4†)	8	1	2	5	3	6	5	3	...
40 mEq Na	5(4†)	8	1	2	5	3	6	5	3	1/4 tsp
90 mEq Na	5†	8†	1	2†	5	3(1†)	6	5	3	1/4 tsp
70 Gram Protein: 85 mEq										
potassium, 2,200 ml fluid										
20 mEq Na	5	6	4	6	...	4	6	6	3	...
40 mEq Na	5(4†)	6†	4	6	...	4	6	6	3	...
90 mEq Na	5†	6†	4	6†	...	4	6	6	3	...
100 Gram Protein: 95 mEq										
potassium, 2,200 ml fluid										
30 mEq Na	9	6	4	6	...	4	5	4	3	...
40 mEq Na	9	6†	4	6	...	4	5	4	3	...
90 mEq Na	9	6†	4	6†	...	4	5	4	3	1/8 tsp
120 Gram Protein: 95 mEq										
potassium, 2,300 ml fluid										
90 mEq Na	11†	6†	6	7	...	3	4	2	3	1/4 tsp

*A half cup of half and half is included in all diets (4 gm protein, 14 gm fat, 6 gm carbohydrate, 165 calories). When other milk products are included, the nutritive composition of the diet should be reevaluated.

†In place of salt allowance, the equivalent in salted foods may be given.

†Foods salted in preparation or processing.

FOOD GROUPS (Values Based on Averages for Food Groups, pages 81–86)

Food	Approximate amount	Protein gm	Calories	Sodium mEq Unsalted	Sodium mEq Salted	Potassium mEq	Fluid ml
Egg	1	7	75	3.0	5.0	2.0	35
Meat	1 ounce	7	75	1.0	3.0*	2.5	20
Fat	Varies	...	35	...	2.0	...	1
Milk Product	Varies	4	Varies	2.5	2.5	4.0	70
Bread	1 slice	2	70	0.5	6.0	1.5	10
Potato	1/2 cup	2	70	0.5	10.0†	7.0	80
Cereal	1/2 cup	2	70	0.5	10.0†	1.5	Varies
Vegetable							
Group 1	Varies	1	20	0.3	10.0†	3.0	60
Group 2	Varies	1	20	0.8	11.0†	5.0	80
(Average value)				(0.5)		(4.0)	(70)
Fruit							
Group 1	Varies	0.5	60	...	...	2.5	80
Group 2	Varies	0.5	60	...	...	5.0	75
(Average value)						(3.0)	(80)
Low Protein Bread	1 slice (40 grams)	0.2	115	0.5	...	0.3	10
CHO Supplement	Varies	...	120	...	...	1.0	Varies
Beverage (coffee, tea)	1 cup	...	...	...	...	2.0	240
Salt	1 teaspoon	...	...	...	86	...	...

*Moderately salted during preparation, approximately 1/2 teaspoon salt per pound of meat.
†Moderately salted during preparation or processing, approximately 1/8 teaspoon of salt per 1/2 cup.

MAYO CLINIC FOOD EXCHANGE LIST FOR DIETS WITH CONTROLLED PROTEIN, SODIUM, AND POTASSIUM

Meat Group (Unsalted)	Protein	7.0 gm
	Sodium	1.0 mEq
	Potassium	2.5 mEq
	Calories	75
	Water	20 ml

	Amount	Weight gm
Meat (unsalted)		
Beef, lamb, liver, pork, veal	1 ounce	30
Fowl (unsalted)		
Chicken, duck, turkey	1 ounce	30
Fish (unsalted — fresh or frozen)		
Fish	1 ounce	30
Clams	2 ounces	50
Oysters	2½ ounces	50
Shrimp	1 ounce	30
Egg (unsalted—3 mEq sodium)	1 medium	50
Cheese (unsalted)		
Cheese	1 ounce	30
Cottage cheese	1/4 cup	50
Peanut Butter (unsalted)	2 tablespoons	30

Omitted: Salted meat, fish, fowl, cheese, peanut butter; other organ meats; other shellfish

Fat Group (Unsalted)	Protein	...
	Sodium	...
	Potassium	...
	Calories	35
	Water	1 ml

	Amount	Weight gm
Margarine	1 teaspoon	5
Mayonnaise	1 teaspoon	5
Cooking fats or oils	1 teaspoon	5

Omitted: Salted butter or margarine; commercial salad dressings

Milk Group	Protein	4.0 gm
	Sodium	2.5 mEq
	Potassium	4.0 mEq
	Calories	Varies
	Water	70 ml

	Amount	Weight gm
Milk	1/2 cup	120
Evaporated or condensed milk	1/4 cup	60
Yogurt	1/2 cup	120
Powdered whole milk	2 tablespoons	14
Half and half (coffee cream)	1/2 cup	120
Light whipping cream	2/3 cup	160
Heavy whipping cream	3/4 cup	180
Sour cream	1/2 cup	120
Ice cream	1/2 cup	100
Ice milk	1/3 cup	80
Sherbet	1 cup	240
Custard	1/4 cup	60

Omitted: Commercial buttermilk, powdered skim milk, instant dairy mixes, nondairy cream substitutes

Bread Group (Unsalted)	Protein	2.0 gm
	Sodium	0.5 mEq
	Potassium	1.5 mEq
	Calories	70
	Water	Varies

	Amount	Weight gm
Bread (unsalted)	1 slice	25
Cereal (unsalted)		
Cooked	1/2 cup	100
Dry, flake	2/3 cup	20
Dry, puffed wheat or rice	1 1/2 cups	20
Dry, biscuit	1	25
Crackers (unsalted)		
Crackers	6	20
Melba toast	4	15
Flour Products (unsalted)		
Flour	2 tablespoons	20
Cornmeal	2 tablespoons	25
Macaroni, noodles, spaghetti		
Dry	1/2 ounce	15
Cooked	1/4 cup	50
Rice		
Dry	1 ounce	30
Cooked	1/2 cup	100

Vegetable (unsalted)

Brussels sprouts	1/4 cup	50
*Corn	1/3 cup	80
Corn grits	1/2 cup	100
Lima beans	1/4 cup	50
*Parsnips	1/2 cup	100
Peas	1/4 cup	50
*Potato	1/2 cup	100
*Sweet potato, fresh or canned	1/2 cup	100

Miscellaneous

Milk or sweet chocolate	1 ounce	30
Pie crust (unsalted)	1/8 pie (9″)	135
Popcorn	1 cup	14

Omitted: Breads, rolls, or crackers made with salt, baking powder, or baking soda; self-rising flour; instant, quick-cooking or ready-to-eat cereals processed with salt or sodium compound; commercially prepared mixes; dried beans or peas, commercially frozen peas

*Potassium—3–9 mEq.

Low Protein Bread Group (Unsalted)	Protein	0.2 gm
	Sodium	0.5 mEq
	Potassium	...
	Calories	115
	Water	10 ml

	Amount	Weight gm

Low Protein Products

	Amount	Weight gm
Bread	1 slice	40
Pasta, cooked	1½ cups	135
Rusk	2 slices	20

Low Protein Bread

	Amount	Weight gm
(made with low protein bread mix)	1 slice	40

Recipes for other low protein products should be calculated individually. Wheat starch, cornstarch, arrowroot, and tapioca may be used in preparation of breads and desserts.

Vegetable Groups (Unsalted)

Group 1	Protein	1.0 gm
	Sodium	0.3 mEq
	Potassium	3.0 mEq*
	Calories	20
	Water	60 ml

Unsalted	Amount	Weight gm
Asparagus, fresh, frozen, canned	1/4 cup	50
Bean sprouts	1/2 cup	50
Beans (green or wax), canned	1/2 cup	100
Broccoli, fresh or frozen	1/4 cup	50
Carrots, canned	1/2 cup	100
†Cauliflower, fresh or frozen	1/4 cup	50
Collards, cooked	1/4 cup	50
Dandelion greens, cooked	1/4 cup	50
†Endive	1/2 cup	50
†Escarole	4 leaves	50

Unsalted	Amount	Weight
		gm
†Lettuce	1/4 small head	100
Mustard greens, cooked	1/4 cup	50
Okra	1/4 cup	50
†Onions	1/2 cup	50
Pepper, green	1/4 cup	50
Radishes	10	100
Rutabaga, fresh or frozen	1/3 cup	80
Spinach, cooked	1/4 cup	50
Squash	1/3 cup	80

*Potassium restrictions: cooked vegetables, drained.
†May be eaten raw in amounts specified.

Group 2	Protein	1.0 gm
	Sodium	0.8 mEq
	Potassium	5.0 mEq*
	Calories	20
	Water	80 ml

Unsalted	Amount	Weight
		gm
Beans (green or wax), fresh or frozen	1/2 cup	100
Beets, fresh, frozen, or canned	1/2 cup	100
†Cabbage, fresh	1/2 cup	100
Carrots, fresh or frozen	1/4 cup	50
†Cucumber	1/2 cup	100
†Eggplant	1/2 cup	100
†Mushrooms, fresh	2 large or 5 small	50
†Pepper, green, fresh	1/3 cup	80
Pumpkin	1/3 cup	80
†Tomato, fresh or canned	1/2 cup or 1 small	100
Tomato juice, canned	1/2 cup	120
Turnip greens, cooked	1/3 cup	80
†Watercress	10 sprigs	50

Omitted: Vegetables processed or prepared with salt, sodium, or sodium compound; any vegetable not listed

*Potassium restrictions: cooked vegetables, drained.
†May be eaten raw in amounts specified.

Fruit Groups

Group 1	Protein	0.5 gm
	Sodium	...
	Potassium	2.5 mEq
	Calories	60
	Water	80 ml

	Amount	Weight
		gm
Apple	1 (2″ diameter)	80
Apple juice	1/2 cup	120
Applesauce	1/2 cup	100
Blackberries	1/4 cup	50
Blueberries	1/2 cup	100
Cantaloupe	1/4 small	50
Cherries, canned or frozen	1/3 cup	80
Coconut, fresh or dried	1/2 ounce	15

	Amount	Weight gm
Cranberries, fresh	1/2 cup	100
Cranberry juice	2 cups	480
Dates	2	15
Grapefruit, fresh	1/2 small	100
Grapefruit sections, canned	1/2 cup	100
Grapes, canned	1/3 cup	80
Grapes, fresh	1/3 cup or 10	50
Grape juice	1/4 cup	60
Grape juice drink	1 cup	240
Honeydew melon	1/4 small	50
Lemon juice	1/2 cup or 1 lemon	100
Loganberries	1/3 cup	80
Mango, fresh	1 medium	70
Orange-apricot drink	1/2 cup	120
Peach, frozen	1/2 cup	100
Peach nectar	2/3 cup	160
Pear, fresh	1 small	80
Pear, canned	3/4 cup	150
Pear nectar	3/4 cup	180
Pineapple, canned	1/2 cup	100
Pineapple, fresh or frozen	1/3 cup	80
Pineapple-grapefruit drink	2/3 cup	160
Pineapple-orange drink	2/3 cup	160
Plums, canned	3	80
Raisins	2 tablespoons	15
Raspberries, frozen	1/3 cup	80
Strawberries, frozen	1/2 cup	100
Tangerine	2 small	80
Watermelon	1/2 cup	100

Group 2   Protein   0.5 gm
Sodium   ...
Potassium   5.0 mEq
Calories   55
Water   75 ml

	Amount	Weight gm
Apricots	1 medium	80
Apricot nectar	1/2 cup	120
Banana, fresh	1/2 small	60
Blackberries, fresh	1/3 cup	80
Figs, canned	1/2 cup	100
Figs, fresh	1 large	50
Fruit cocktail, canned	1/2 cup	100
Grapefruit juice	1/2 cup	120
Melon balls, frozen	1/3 cup	80
Nectarines, fresh	1 small	80
Orange, fresh	1 small	80
Orange juice, fresh, frozen, or canned	1/2 cup	120
Papaya, fresh	1/3 cup	80
Peaches, fresh or canned	2 halves	100
Persimmon, fresh	1/2 small	60
Pineapple juice	1/2 cup	120
Plums, fresh	2 small	80

	Amount	Weight
		gm
Prune juice	1/2 cup	120
Prunes	2 small	15
Raspberries	1/3 cup	80
Rhubarb	1/3 cup	80
Strawberries, fresh	1/2 cup	100

Omitted: Any fruit not listed

Carbohydrate Supplement Group (CHO Supplement)	Protein	...
	Sodium	...
	Potassium	1 mEq
	Calories	120
	Water	Varies

	Amount	Weight
		gm
Sugar and syrups		
Sugar	2½ tablespoons	30
Honey	2 tablespoons	40
Jelly or jam	2 tablespoons	40
Syrup (table blends)	2 tablespoons	40
Candy		
Fondant or sugar mints	3	30
Gumdrops	3 large	30
Hard candy, unfilled	6 pieces	30
Jelly beans	20	60
Lollipops, unfilled	1 medium	30
Fruit desserts		
Cranberry (sauce or relish)	2 tablespoons	80
Fruit ice	⅔ cup	140
Popsicle	1 twin bar	130
Flavored beverages (carbonated, fruit flavored, Kool Aid, lemonade)	1 cup (8 ounces)	240
Flour products		
Cornstarch or tapioca	¼ cup	30

Beverage (Values Should Be Calculated Individually)

	Amount	Weight	Potassium
		gm	mEq
Coffee, tea	1 cup	240	2

Miscellaneous

Allowed	Omitted
Pepper; spices and herbs except "Omitted," fresh celery (no more than 2 tablespoons); fresh garlic, onion powder or juice; horseradish root, powdered mustard; vinegar; unsalted white sauce made with milk allowance; flavoring extracts	Salt,* seasoned salts, mixed spices; baking powder, baking soda; parsley, dried celery products; bottled meat sauces, catsup, prepared mustard or horseradish, meat extracts, meat tenderizers, monosodium glutamate; pickles; gravy; commercial soups; commercially prepared dessert mixes; cocoa; nuts; olives; salt substitutes unless approved by physician

*Allowed when specifically calculated.

PREOPERATIVE AND POSTOPERATIVE DIETARY PROGRAMS

MODIFIED RESIDUE DIETS

Minimum Residue Diet; Restricted Residue Diet

NUTRITIONAL ADEQUACY

The Minimum Residue Diet may be inadequate in B vitamins and minerals according to the Recommended Daily Dietary Allowances of the National Research Council. The physician may wish to prescribe supplements if the diet is followed for an extended time.

The Restricted Residue Diet meets the recommended nutrient levels according to the Recommended Daily Dietary Allowances of the National Research Council.

APPROXIMATE COMPOSITION (10 to 15% Variation)

Diet	Protein gm	Fat gm	Carbohydrate gm	Calories	Sodium* mEq	Potassium mEq	Fluid ml
Minimum Residue	70	90	230	2,010	115	60	1,600
Restricted Residue	70	95	230	2,055	110	80	2,000

*Value is for average amount of salt used in preparation of foods; salt added to food at the table is not calculated.

GENERAL INFORMATION

The Modified Residue Diets consist of foods believed to produce minimal or moderate residue in the gastrointestinal tract. The physician should specify the level of residue desired, either **minimum** or **restricted**, when ordering a modified residue diet. Diets available are as follows:

Minimum Residue.   The diet is severely restricted in residue-producing foods. It may be ordered when the gastrointestinal tract is to be as clear of undigested foods as possible. Whole fruits and vegetables are omitted and dairy products are limited to cottage cheese and mild cheese used as flavoring. A small amount of milk or half and half is allowed.

Restricted Residue.   The diet is moderately restricted in residue. It may be ordered as a postoperative diet for patients who are unable to tolerate the amount of residue in the general diet. Foods with a small amount of fiber, such as canned or cooked fruits and vegetables, are allowed. Milk or milk products should be limited to two cups or less per day.

The Modified Residue Diets are planned with the Mayo Clinic Food Exchange List. Servings of food exchanges are suggested in the following table. This table should be used only as a guide in planning the diets. Modifications within the prescribed dietary restrictions may be made in order to adapt the diet to the normal dietary pattern of the hospital or the patient.

SUGGESTED DAILY FOOD EXCHANGES (Mayo Clinic Food Exchange List, inside covers)

Diet	Meat*	Fat*	Milk	Bread*	Vegetable	Fruit	Dessert*	Sweets*
Minimum Residue	7	10[†]	...[†]	8	2 (juice)	2 (juice)	2	4
Restricted Residue	5	9	2	6	3	2	2	4

*Amounts not restricted.
†One half cup of half and half or other milk product may be used per day.

SUGGESTED MENU PATTERN

	Minimum Residue Diet	Restricted Residue Diet
Breakfast		
Fruit	1 serving*	1 serving
Egg	1	1
Cereal	1 serving	1 serving
Bread	1 slice	1 slice
Fat	4 teaspoons	3 teaspoons
Sugar, jelly	2 tablespoons	2 tablespoons
Beverage	1 cup	1 cup
Noon Meal		
Meat	3 ounces	2 ounces
Potato	1 serving†	1 serving
Vegetable	1 serving*	1 serving
Salad	...	1 serving
Bread	2 slices	1 slice
Fat	3 teaspoons	3 teaspoons
Dessert	1 serving	1 serving
Milk	...	1 cup
Sugar, jelly	1 tablespoon	1 tablespoon
Beverage	1 cup	1 cup
Evening Meal		
Meat	3 ounces	2 ounces
Potato	1 serving†	1 serving
Vegetable	1 serving*	1 serving
Salad	...	1 serving
Bread	2 slices	1 slice
Fat	3 teaspoons	3 teaspoons
Dessert	1 serving	1 serving
Milk	...	1 cup
Sugar, jelly	1 tablespoon	1 tablespoon
Beverage	1 cup	1 cup

*Juice.
†Potato substitute.

FOOD GROUPS

Minimum Residue Diet

Allowed	*Omitted*
	Fried and highly seasoned foods
Beverage	
Coffee, tea; carbonated beverage; cereal beverage	
Meat	
Meat, fish, or fowl; egg; cottage cheese, mild cheese as flavoring; cream style peanut butter	Fried; meat or shellfish with tough connective tissue; other cheese
Fat	
Any except "Omitted"; half and half, 1/2 cup or less per day	Avocado; olives; nuts; highly seasoned salad dressings
Milk	
One half cup of milk may be used in place of cream allowance	
Bread	
Refined wheat or rye bread, rolls, or crackers	Any with whole grain or graham flour, bran, seeds or nuts; quick breads
Refined cereals — cooked or ready to eat; strained oatmeal	Whole grain or bran cereals
Macaroni, noodles, refined rice, spaghetti	Potato; whole grain rice; dried legumes; corn, lima beans, peas; popcorn; hominy
Vegetable	
Mild-flavored vegetable juice	Whole vegetables
Fruit	
Fruit juice, strained	Whole fruit
Soup	
Bouillon, broth	Any other
Dessert	
Cake, cookies; gelatin; sherbet, ice cream; puddings (note milk allowance)	Any with coconut, nuts, or whole fruit; pastries
Sweets	
Any except "Omitted"	Jam, marmalade; candy with coconut, nuts, or whole fruit
Miscellaneous	
Salt, spices, and herbs except "Omitted"; vinegar; gravy, white sauce; chocolate	Garlic; seed spices; pickles; condiments; cocoa mixes

FOOD GROUPS

Restricted Residue Diet

Allowed	Omitted
Beverage	
Coffee, tea; carbonated beverage; cereal beverage	
Meat	
Meat, fish, or fowl; egg; cottage cheese, mild cheese as flavoring; cream style peanut butter	Meat or shellfish with tough connective tissue, other cheese
Fat	
Any except "Omitted"	Avocado; nuts; olives
Milk	
Milk, milk drinks: no more than 2 cups per day	
Bread	
Refined wheat or rye bread, rolls, or crackers	Any with whole grain or graham flour, bran, seeds or nuts; quick breads
Refined cereals — cooked or ready to eat	Whole grain or bran cereals
Potato and potato substitutes except "Omitted"; hominy grits; puréed corn, lima beans, peas	Whole grain rice; dried legumes; popcorn
Vegetable	
Canned or cooked mild-flavored vegetables without seed or coarse fiber; lettuce, tomatoes (no seeds or skins)	Any other
Fruit	
Canned or cooked fruits without seeds or tough skin; fruit juice; banana; citrus fruits without membrane	Any other
Soup	
Broth, bouillon; soup with "Allowed" foods	Any other
Dessert	
Any except "Omitted"	Any with coconut, nuts, or "Omitted" fruits
Sweets	
Any except "Omitted"	Jam, marmalade; candy with coconut, nuts, or "Omitted" fruits
Miscellaneous	
Salt; spices and herbs except "Omitted"; condiments (as tolerated); chocolate, cocoa; gravy, white sauce; vinegar	Garlic, seed spices; pickles

DIETARY REGIMENS FOR SURGICAL PATIENTS

GENERAL POSTOPERATIVE DIETARY REGIMEN

The general postoperative dietary regimen can be ordered after most surgical procedures. The surgeon may indicate specific dietary restrictions on the Hospital Diet Request Form. The following options are available:

Dietary progression	Duration and advancement	Dietary regimen*
Slow	4 days	
	1st day	Clear Liquid
	2nd day	Full Liquid
	3rd day	Soft
	4th day	General
Regular	3 days	
	1st day	Clear Liquid to Full Liquid
	2nd day	Soft
	3rd day	General
Rapid	1 day	
	1st day	Clear Liquid to General by 3rd meal

*See Section on Standard Hospital Diets, pages 6 to 11.

SPECIAL POSTOPERATIVE DIETARY REGIMEN

Special dietary regimens are indicated after the following categories of surgical procedures: cardiac, esophageal, gastric, and plastic and laryngeal.

Cardiac Surgery.   A dietary regimen that contains either 20 mEq or less of sodium or 90 mEq or less of sodium may be ordered.

Diet*	Duration and advancement		Dietary regimen†
20 mEq or Less of Sodium	3 days		
	1st day	Clear Liquid	
	2nd day	Full Liquid	20 mEq or less sodium
	3rd day	General	
90 mEq or Less of Sodium	3 days		
	1st day	Clear Liquid	
	2nd day	Full Liquid	90 mEq or less sodium
	3rd day	General	

*See Sodium-Restricted Diets, pages 22 to 25.
†See Standard Hospital Diets, pages 6 to 11.

Esophageal Surgery.   A dietary regimen with or without liberal ulcer features may be ordered.

Diet*	Duration and advancement	Dietary regimen†
Standard Hospital Diets with Liberal Ulcer Features	3 days 1st day 2nd day 3rd day	Clear Liquid Full Liquid Mechanically soft Liberal Ulcer
Standard Hospital Diets Without Ulcer Features	3 days 1st day 2nd day 3rd day	Clear Liquid Full Liquid Mechanically soft

*See Standard Hospital Diets, pages 6 to 11.
†See Liberal Ulcer Diet, pages 39, 40, and 45

Gastric Resection.   After gastric resection the following dietary regimen may be ordered when the patient is able to tolerate food.

Diet*	Duration	Dietary regimen
Standard Hospital Diets: Clear Liquid Full Liquid Soft General	5 days	Diet as ordered served in **6 small feedings.** Number of feedings to be decreased as tolerated

*See Standard Hospital Diets, pages 6 to 11.

For patients who may experience "dumping syndrome" after gastric resection, a dry diet may be ordered. The diet should be high in protein (100 to 120 gm) and low in carbohydrate (100 to 125 gm), with fat as tolerated for additional calories. Fluids may be taken 1 hour before or after meals.

Plastic and Laryngeal Surgery.   After oral or laryngeal operations, the following dietary regimens may be ordered.

Diet

Full Liquid with Funnel
   Liquids that will pass through a funnel

Full Liquid Without Funnel
   Food similar to that served on the Full Liquid Diet

Soft Diet
   Soft and puréed foods as tolerated by the patient

Tube Feedings
   Standard, Blenderized, or Commercial Feedings, pages 94 and 95.

TUBE FEEDINGS

STANDARD, BLENDERIZED, AND COMMERCIAL FEEDINGS

Standard Tube Feeding

NUTRITIONAL ADEQUACY

The Standard Tube Feeding (1,500 ml) may be inadequate in iron for men and women.

APPROXIMATE COMPOSITION (10 to 15% Variation)

Protein	Fat	Carbohydrate	Calories*	Sodium	Potassium	Fluid
gm	gm	gm		mEq	mEq	ml
100	110	190	2,140	155	100	1,500

*1.4 calories per milliliter.

GENERAL INFORMATION

The Standard Tube Feeding is a milk-base tube feeding to which eggnog powder and a vitamin preparation are added. This feeding contains approximately 1.4 calories per milliliter. The formula may be diluted if it is not tolerated at this concentration.

The physician should order the total amount of tube feeding needed in 24 hours. The amount given at one time may vary from 150 to 200 ml.

Modifications may be made when variations in one or more nutrients are necessary. Orders for any tube feedings other than the Standard Tube Feeding should specify the desired amounts of protein, fat, carbohydrate, calories, or other nutrients (sodium, potassium) to be modified.

Ingredients	Weight	Approximate amount
	gm	
Milk, whole	800	3 1/3 cups
Eggnog powder	100	2/3 cup
Skim milk, powdered	90	3/4 cup
Half and half	600	2 1/2 cups
Salt	5.5	1 teaspoon
Vitamin preparation*	5	1 1/4 teaspoons
Water to 1,500 ml		

Preparation: Combine ingredients in an electric mixer, mix well, and refrigerate.

*The vitamin supplement (5 ml) contains 2 mg of thiamine, 3 mg of riboflavin, 30 mg of niacin, and 100 mg of ascorbic acid.

Blenderized Tube Feeding

APPROXIMATE COMPOSITION (10 to 15% Variation)

Protein	Fat	Carbohydrate	Calories*	Sodium	Potassium	Fluid
gm	gm	gm		mEq	mEq	ml
150	60	230	2,050	100	143	1,500

*1.3 calories per milliliter.

GENERAL INFORMATION

The Blenderized Tube Feeding is prepared from a variety of basic foods; these foods are mixed in a blender and strained. Foods from the general diet such as meat, fruits, vegetables, eggnog powder, and milk products are used. The tube feeding contains approximately 1.3 calories per milliliter.

The physician should order the total amount needed in 24 hours. The amount of tube feeding given at one time may be from 150 to 200 ml.

Ingredients	Weight	Approximate amount
	gm	
Meat, strained	210	1 cup
Eggnog powder	75	1/2 cup
Vegetable, strained	120	1/2 cup
Fruit juice	240	1 cup
Milk, whole	720	3 cups
Skim milk, powdered	180	2 cups
Half and half	150	5/8 cup
Water to make 1,500 ml		

Preparation: Combine ingredients in an electric mixer or blender. Mix well and strain if necessary. Refrigerate.

Commercial Feedings

Various commercially prepared feedings are available. If necessary, commercial feedings may be ordered.

TEST DIETS

120 MILLIGRAM CALCIUM TEST DIET (700 MILLIGRAMS PHOSPHORUS)

APPROXIMATE COMPOSITION

Protein	Fat	Carbohydrate	Calories	Calcium	Phosphorus
gm	gm	gm		mg	mg
60	102	235	2,050	120	700

GENERAL INFORMATION

This diet is a low calcium diet similar to that of Bauer and Aub.[*]

The diet may be ordered for treatment of acute hypercalcemia or as a test diet for diagnosis of hypercalciuria. The diet should be used for a limited time only, as it is low in calcium.

When used as a diagnostic measure, the diet should be followed for 3 days. Water for cooking or drinking should be distilled water. The patient should receive his meals either in the hospital or at a special "diet kitchen."

---

[*]Bauer, W., and Aub, J. C.: Studies of inorganic salt metabolism. I. The ward routine and methods. J. Amer. Diet. Ass. *3:*106–115 (Sept.) 1927.

MENU PATTERN

	Weight *gm*	Approximate amount
Breakfast		
Orange juice	100	1/2 cup
with sugar	10	2 1/2 teaspoons
Farina, cooked	140	2/3 cup
Soda crackers	20	5
Butter	25	5 teaspoons
Bacon	15	3 strips
Sugar, jelly	14	1 tablespoon
Beverage*		
Noon Meal		
Meat[†]	75	2 1/2 ounces
Potato, boiled or baked	100	1/2 cup
Tomato, raw or canned	100	1 small
Soda crackers	20	5
Butter	25	5 teaspoons
Fruit[†]	100	1 serving
Sugar, jelly	14	1 tablespoon
Beverage*		
Evening Meal		
Meat[†]	75	2 1/2 ounces
Rice, cooked	100	1/2 cup
Corn	100	1/2 cup
Soda crackers	20	5
Butter	25	5 teaspoons
Fruit[†]	100	1 serving
Sugar, jelly	14	1 tablespoon
Beverage*		

*Coffee or tea made with distilled water may be served.
†Beef, lamb, veal, or chicken may be used.
†Applesauce (½ cup), 1 banana, 1 peach, or 1 small slice of watermelon may be used.

700 MILLIGRAM CALCIUM TEST DIET

APPROXIMATE COMPOSITION (10 to 15 % Variation)

Protein	Fat	Carbohydrate	Calories	Calcium	Phosphorus
gm	gm	gm		mg	mg
70	95	230	2,055	710	1,030

GENERAL INFORMATION

The diet is used for *1 day only* in the diagnosis of hypercalciuria unless the physician indicates otherwise. The diet may be served in a "diet kitchen" or in the hospital. If the diet is to be followed at home, the patient should be instructed in the dietary program.

The 700 Milligram Calcium Test Diet is planned with the Mayo Clinic Food Exchange List. Servings of food exchanges are given in the following table. The amount of food and fluid listed should not be modified.

DAILY FOOD EXCHANGES (Mayo Clinic Food Exchange List, inside covers)

Meat	Fat	Milk	Bread	Vegetable	Fruit	Dessert	Sweets	Fluid
6	11*	1	7	4	2	1	4	6–8 cups†

*One half cup of half and half daily.
†Daily water intake (including coffee or tea) should be between 1,440 and 1,920 ml.

Foods Omitted

Meat
Fish, shellfish; cheese; peanut butter

Soup
Cream soup or any made with foods not allowed

Bread
Whole grain bread or cereals; dried peas and beans

Dessert
Ice cream, ice milk, puddings, custard or any made with chocolate, milk, or nuts

Vegetable
Leafy, dark green vegetables

Sweets
Candy made with chocolate, milk, or nuts

Fruit
Dried fruit

Miscellaneous
Chocolate, cocoa

SUGGESTED MENU PATTERN

Breakfast

Fruit	1/2 cup
Egg	1
Cereal, corn or rice (dry)	1 cup
Half and half	1/2 cup
Bread	2 slices
Fat	3 teaspoons
Beverage*	1 cup
Sugar, jelly	2 tablespoons

Noon Meal

Meat or fowl	2 ounces
Potato, baked or boiled	1 serving
Vegetable	1 serving
Salad	1 serving
Bread	1 slice
Fat	2 teaspoons
Fruit	1 serving
Milk	1 cup
Beverage*	1 cup
Sugar, jelly	1 tablespoon

Evening Meal

Meat or fowl	3 ounces
Potato, baked or boiled	1 serving
Vegetable	1 serving
Salad	1 serving
Bread	1 slice
Fat	2 teaspoons
Dessert	1 serving
Beverage*	1 cup
Sugar, jelly	1 tablespoon

*Daily water intake (including coffee or tea) should be between 1,440 and 1,920 ml.

100 GRAM FAT TEST DIET[1]

APPROXIMATE COMPOSITION * (10 to 15% Variation)

Protein	Fat	Carbohydrate	Calories	Sodium*	Potassium	Fluid
gm	*gm*	*gm*		*mEq*	*mEq*	*ml*
120	100	270	2,460	100	100	2,500

*Average values for three menu patterns, page 101; values calculated by chemical analyses.
†Value is for average amount of salt used in preparation of foods; salt added to food at the table is not calculated.

GENERAL INFORMATION

The diet, which is used in the diagnosis of steatorrhea or azotorrhea, is given for 3 days unless otherwise indicated. The physician should order the test diet only for a patient who can eat in a "diet kitchen" or who is hospitalized during the test period.

The dietary regimen consists of three menus to be served during the test period. All food should be weighed. The amount and kind of food specified on the menus should not be modified. The diet includes between-meal feedings of high calorie milk beverage.

---

[1]Wollaeger, E. E., Comfort, M. W., and Osterberg, A. E.: Total solids, fat and nitrogen in the feces. III. A study of normal persons taking a test diet containing a moderate amount of fat; Comparison with results obtained with normal persons taking a test diet containing a large amount of fat. Gastroenterology *9:*272-283 (Sept.) 1947.

MENU PATTERNS FOR THREE DAYS

First day	Weight gm	Second day	Weight gm	Third day	Weight gm
Breakfast					
Orange juice	100	Pineapple juice	100	Orange juice	100
Rice Krispies	14	Cream of Wheat	14	Malt-o-Meal	14
Eggs (2)	100	Egg (1)	50	Egg (1)	50
White toast	40	White toast	40	White toast	40
Butter	10	Butter	10	Butter	10
Whole milk	200	Whole milk	200	Whole milk	200
Honey or jelly	25	Honey or jelly	25	Honey or jelly	25
Sugar	7	Sugar	7	Sugar	7
Coffee or tea, if desired		Coffee or tea, if desired		Coffee or tea, if desired	
Noon Meal					
Lean beef or lamb, raw weight	75	Lean beef or lamb, raw weight	75	Lean beef or lamb, raw weight	75
Potato	50	Potato	50	Potato	50
Tomato juice	100	Carrots	50	Green beans	50
Salad: sliced apple and lettuce	50 / 10	Salad: pineapple and lettuce	50 / 10	Salad: deviled egg (1) and lettuce	50 / 10
Apricots	80	Custard: milk and egg (1)	100 / 50	Fruit cup: orange, pineapple, and pear	50 / 25 / 25
White bread	20	White bread	20	White bread	20
Butter	10	Butter	10	Butter	10
Whole milk	200	Whole milk	200	Whole milk	200
Evening Meal					
Lean beef, raw weight	75	Lean beef, raw weight	75	Lean beef, raw weight	75
Cooked rice	50	Cooked spaghetti	50	Potato	50
Canned peas	50	Tomato juice	50	Beets	50
Salad: prune and lettuce	50 / 10	Salad: flavored gelatin and Royal Ann cherries	65 / 50	Salad: pears, jelly, and lettuce	50 / 20 / 10
Peaches	65	Baked apple	100	Bing cherries	50
White bread	20	Sugar	7	White bread	20
Butter	6	White bread	20	Butter	6
Whole milk	200	Butter	6	Whole milk	200
		Whole milk	200		
Between-Meal Feedings (for the day)					
Whole milk	600	Whole milk	600	Whole milk	600
Dietene	60	Dietene	60	Dietene	60

RENIN TEST DIET

APPROXIMATE COMPOSITION (10 to 15% Variation)

Protein	Fat	Carbohydrate	Calories	Sodium*	Potassium	Fluid
gm	gm	gm		mEq	mEq	ml
60	85	225	1,900	20	90	1,700

*Ten milliequivalents sodium test diet may be ordered.

GENERAL INFORMATION

The test diet is used in the investigation of patients with renovascular, renal, or primary hypertension. The physician should specify the number of days that the diet should be followed.

Foods included in the test diet are prepared with tap water. If the physician orders a 10 mEq sodium test diet, distilled water is used.

Foods are prepared or processed without salt. The Renin Test Diet is planned with the Mayo Clinic Food Exchange List. Servings of food exchanges and beverages listed in the following table should not be modified. Distilled water is the only fluid allowed between meals.

DAILY FOOD EXCHANGES* (Mayo Clinic Food Exchange List, inside covers)

Meat	Fat	Milk	Bread	Vegetable	Fruit	Sweets	Coffee
6	12†	†	7	4	4	4	3 cups

*Amounts as indicated.
†One half cup of half and half or other dairy product may be used daily.

SUGGESTED MENU PATTERN*

	Weight	Approximate amount
	gm	
Breakfast		
Orange juice, fresh	240	1 cup
Egg	50	1
Cereal (dry)	20	Varies
Half and half	120	1/2 cup
Bread	50	2 slices
Fat	10	2 teaspoons
Coffee	240	1 cup
Sugar, jelly (as desired)		
Noon Meal		
Meat, cooked	60	2 ounces
Potato	100	1/2 cup
Tomato juice	100	1/2 cup
Vegetable	100	1/2 cup
Bread	25	1 slice
Fat	15	3 teaspoons
Fruit	120	1/2 cup
Coffee	240	1 cup
Sugar, jelly (as desired)		

Evening Meal

Meat, cooked	90	3 ounces
Potato	100	1/2 cup
Vegetable	100	1/2 cup
Bread	25	1 slice
Fat	15	3 teaspoons
Fruit	120	1/2 cup
Coffee	240	1 cup
Sugar, jelly (as desired)		

*Foods processed or prepared without salt.

SECTION 4

STANDARD HOSPITAL DIETS FOR CHILDREN

GENERAL HOSPITAL DIETS

NUTRITIONAL ADEQUACY

The Recommended Daily Dietary Allowances of the National Research Council are used as guides in planning hospital diets for children. Because of reduced activity, the number of calories in hospital diets for children may be lower than the recommended allowances.

The physician may wish to prescribe vitamin and mineral supplements when specific deficiencies need to be corrected.

APPROXIMATE COMPOSITION (10 to 15% Variation)

Age years	Protein gm	Fat gm	Carbohydrate gm	Calories*	Sodium† mEq	Potassium mEq	Fluid ml
Less than 2	45	50	100	1,030	50	55	1,100
2 to 6	55	60	120	1,240	70	60	1,200
6 to 14	65	75	170	1,615	90	75	1,400

*Calories are adapted to the age, appetite, and activity of the hospitalized child.
†Amount of salt used in preparation of food; salt added to food at the table is not calculated.

GENERAL INFORMATION

A description of suggested foods and diet patterns for hospitalized children up to 14 years of age follows.

Less Than 1 Year of Age.   The physician may prescribe vitamins A, C, and D.[1] Additions of puréed or strained foods are offered according to the infant's readiness. A guide for the introduction of new foods is suggested below.

Months
1 to 2	Prepared cereal
2 to 3	Fruits and vegetables, puréed or strained; juice; banana
4 to 5	Meat, puréed or strained; hard cooked egg yolk
6 to 7	Toast, crackers, zwieback; potato; custard, plain puddings, and cookies
8 to 9	Bacon
12	Egg, whole

1 to 2 Years.   Chopped fruits, vegetables, and meats are offered in place of puréed and strained foods if the child displays such readiness. The transition from baby food to the General Hospital Diet for children may occur between the ages of 13 months to 2 years. The size of each serving is adapted to the age, appetite, and activity of the hospitalized child.

2 to 6 Years.   The diet is planned for the child who can tolerate whole foods. Occasionally a child may require diced meats. Food similar to that served on the general menu of the hospital is served. Modifications are made such as removal of fine bones from fish and avoidance of nuts and

---
[1]A fluoride preparation may be indicated if the child resides in an area where the local water supply contains a suboptimal level of fluorine.

fruits with pits or seeds. Sizes of servings are adapted to the age, appetite, and activity of the hospitalized child.

6 to 14 Years.   After the age of 6 years, most foods on the general menu of the hospital may be served. Sizes of servings are adapted to the age, appetite, and activity of the hospitalized child.

The General Hospital Diets for Children are planned with the Mayo Clinic Food Exchange List. Servings of food exchanges are suggested that will supply the protein, mineral, and vitamin requirements for children.   If an increase in calories is required, additional servings of basic foods preferred by the child may be included in the diet.   Because it is of primary importance that the calorie intake of the child be adequate, consideration should be given to food preferences. Usually the hospitalized child does not require the number of calories recommended for a healthy active child.

SUGGESTED DAILY FOOD EXCHANGES* (Mayo Clinic Food Exchange List, inside covers)

Age years	Meat	Fat	Milk†	Bread	Vegetable	Fruit	Dessert
Less than 2	2	2	3	2	1-2	2	...
2 to 6	3	2	3	3	2-3	2-3	1
6 and older	4	3	3	5	3-4	2-3	1

*Additional foods as desired for children requiring higher calorie diets.
†Milk with a reduced fat content may be substituted for whole milk at the discretion of the physician. The amount of milk should not exceed 1 quart per day; a greater quantity may hinder intake of other essential foods.

SUGGESTED MENU PATTERN

	2-year-old*	4-year-old*	8-year-old†
	Approximate amount		
Breakfast			
Fruit	1 serving	1 serving	1 serving
Egg	(optional)	1	1
Cereal	1 serving	1 serving	1 serving
Toast	1/2 slice	1/2 slice	1 slice
Fat	1/2 teaspoon	1/2 teaspoon	1 teaspoon
Milk	1 cup	1 cup	1 cup
Sugar, jelly (optional)			
Noon Meal			
Meat	1 ounce	1 ounce	2 ounces
Potato	1 serving	1 serving	1 serving
Vegetable	1 serving	1 serving	1 serving
Salad	...	1 serving	1 serving
Bread	1/2 slice	1/2 slice	1 slice
Fat	1/2 teaspoon	1/2 teaspoon	1 teaspoon
Milk	1 cup	1 cup	1 cup
Dessert (optional)			
Evening Meal			
Meat	1 ounce	1 ounce	1 ounce
Potato (optional)			
Vegetable	1 serving	1 serving	1 serving
Salad (optional)			
Bread	1/2 slice	1 slice	1 slice
Fat	1 teaspoon	1 teaspoon	1 teaspoon
Fruit	1 serving	1 serving	1 serving
Milk	1 cup	1 cup	1 cup

*Size servings are usually one half the size of portions for adult patients.
†Coffee or tea if physician permits.

MODIFICATIONS OF GENERAL DIETS

GENERAL INFORMATION

For children the physician may order hospital diets with restricted features. Diets for adults may be modified to meet the nutritional requirements of children. Such diets are individualized according to the child's age, appetite, and activity. The following diets are available on request:

Soft Diet.   This diet, which is similar to the Soft Diet for adults (pages 7 and 8), is modified according to the child's tolerances.

Clear Liquid and Full Liquid Diets.   These diets are similar to Clear Liquid or Full Liquid diets for adults (pages 9 to 11) but are modified according to the child's tolerances.

Other diets with therapeutic modifications specifically planned for children are as follows: Diabetic Diets (pages 110 to 113), Ketogenic Diets (pages 114 to 122), and Sodium-Restricted Diets (pages 123 to 127).

Diabetic Diets

APPROXIMATE COMPOSITION (10 to 15% Variation)

Approximate Calories	Protein gm	Fat gm	Carbohydrate gm	Sodium mEq	Potassium mEq	Fluid ml
1,200	50	60	120	65	65	1,300
1,400	60	70	130	80	70	1,400
1,600	70	80	145	90	75	1,400
1,800	80	90	170	115	90	1,500
2,000	85	95	195	125	90	1,500
2,200	100	110	210	135	105	1,600
2,400	110	120	220	145	110	1,600
2,600	115	135	230	155	115	1,900
2,800	125	140	260	165	130	2,000
3,000	130	150	285	185	135	2,000

GENERAL INFORMATION

The diabetic diets for children are weighed diets unless the physician specifies a nonweighed diet. The Mayo Clinic Food Exchange List (inside covers) is used in planning the diets. The Mayo Clinic Food Exchange List was developed from a method adopted by the American Diabetes Association, the U.S. Public Health Service, and the American Dietetic Association. Patterns have been established for diets from 1,200 to 3,000 calories.

The diets for children less than 6 years of age are planned with midmorning, midafternoon, and bedtime feedings. The diets for children 6 years of age and older are planned with midafternoon and bedtime feedings. A midmorning feeding may be included if the physician feels it is necessary. A protein food should be included in each between-meal feeding.

The Basic Four Food Groups (page 3) were used as a guide in planning diabetic diets for children. Because nutritional requirements vary with the age of the child, the nutrient content of a diet should be assessed with the allowances recommended by the National Research Council for the child's age. The diet for a child must be readjusted at least once a year because of changing nutritional needs during the growing period.

The dietitian will calculate the carbohydrate value of all food refused by diabetic patients. Food replacement is given to patients receiving insulin or an oral agent when the carbohydrate value of food refused exceeds 25 gm per meal.

Diabetic diets ordered with additional dietary modifications follow the general pattern of the standard diabetic diets. Modified diabetic diets for children are planned with the Mayo Clinic Food Exchange List.

The postoperative dietary program for diabetic children follows the general pattern of the surgical dietary regimen. Foods allowed in the Clear Liquid, Full Liquid, and Soft diets, with the exception of sugar, are served. The patient progresses to the prescribed diabetic diet as soon as it can be tolerated.

METHOD FOR DETERMINING CALORIE LEVEL

The physician prescribes the calorie level of the diet by selecting a percentage increment in calories above the basal requirements. Percentage increments above basal calories for children may range from 50 to 100%.

Child Less Than 5 Years of Age.
1. The ideal weight of the child is computed according to the Standard Height-Weight-Age

Tables, pages 152 to 157. To determine ideal weight, the actual height and age of the child to the nearest half or full year should be used.

2. The basal calorie requirement is computed by multiplying the ideal weight by the basal calories per pound suggested in the following table.

Basal Calorie Requirements per Pound

Age	Calories per pound	
	Boys	Girls
6 months	25.0	25.0
1 year	25.5	25.5
2 years	25.0	24.5
3 years	23.5	23.5
4 years	23.0	22.0

3. The total number of calories is determined by the addition of the percentage increment to the basal calories. The calorie level of the diet should be within 100 calories of the caloric requirements. Three between-meal feedings are included in the diet pattern.

A sample determination of a diabetic diet follows:

Patient: $3\frac{1}{2}$-year-old girl

      Height: 3 feet 2 inches

      Weight: Actual—25 pounds; ideal—31 pounds (see page 155)

Diet order: Basal calories plus 100%

	Calories
Basal calories for 31 pounds (31×22.75)	705
100% increment of basal calorie requirement	705
Total calories	1,410

The suggested diet pattern, page 110, which may be used in planning the diet should be to the nearest 100 calories (1,400 Calorie Diet).

Child 5 to 14 Years of Age.   1. The ideal weight is computed according to the Standard Height-Weight-Age Tables, pages 152 to 157. To determine ideal weight, the actual height and age of the child to the nearest half or full year shoud be used.

2. The basal calorie requirements and the percentage increment above basal calories is computed according to the directions on the food nomogram, page 160. The calorie level of the diet should be within 100 calories of the total calorie requirement. Midafternoon and bedtime feedings are included in the diet pattern.

A sample determination of a diabetic diet follows:

Patient: 8-year-old boy

      Height: 4 feet 3 inches

      Weight: Actual—55 pounds; ideal—60 pounds (see page 152)

Diet order: Basal calories plus 80%

	Calories
Basal calories for 60 pounds	1,240
80% increment of basal calorie requirement	992
Total calories	2,232

The suggested diet pattern, page 110, which may be followed in planning the diet should be to the nearest 100 calories (2,200 Calorie Diet).

SUGGESTED DIETARY PATTERNS

Servings of food exchanges from the Mayo Clinic Food Exchange List for diabetic diets for children are suggested in the following table. This table should be used only as a guide in planning the diets. Modifications within the prescribed dietary restrictions may be made in order to adapt the diet to the normal dietary pattern of the hospital or the patient. Consideration should be given to the food preferences of the child.

SUGGESTED DAILY FOOD EXCHANGES (Mayo Clinic Food Exchange List, inside covers)

Diet	Meat	Fat	Milk	Bread	Vegetable B*	Fruit
1,200	3	3	3	3	1	3
1,400	4	4	3	4	1	3
1,600	5	5	3	5	1	3
1,800	6	6	3	7	1	3
2,000	6	7	3	9	1	3
2,200	8	8	3	9	1	4
2,400	9	9	3	10	1	4
2,600	9	10	4	10	1	4
2,800	10	10	4	11	1	5
3,000	10	12	4	13	1	5

*Vegetable A Food Group may be included in ordinary amounts with each meal.

SUGGESTED MENU PATTERNS

**Diabetic Diet for a 3 1/2-Year-Old Child
and an 8-Year-Old Child**

	1,400 Calorie Diet (3 1/2-year-old child)	2,200 Calorie Diet (8-year-old child)
	Number of exchanges	
Breakfast		
Fruit	1	1
Egg	1	1
Bread	1	2
Fat	1	2
Milk	1/2	1/2
Midmorning Feeding		
Milk	1/2	...
Noon Meal		
Meat	1	3
Bread	1	2
Fat	1	2
Vegetable A	1	1
Fruit	1	1
Milk	1/2	1
Midafternoon Feeding		
Milk	1/2	1/2
Bread	1/2	1
Fat	1	1
Fruit	...	1
Evening Meal		
Meat	2	3
Bread	1	2
Fat	1	2
Vegetable A	Optional	Optional
Vegetable B	1	1
Fruit	1	1
Milk	1/2	1/2
Bedtime		
Milk	1/2	1/2
Meat	...	1
Bread	1/2	2
Fat	...	1

Ketogenic Diet for Children

GENERAL INFORMATION

The ketogenic diet is a weighed diet used in the prophylactic treatment of some types of epilepsy in children. The diet is planned to produce ketosis by reversing the ratio of protein and carbohydrate to fat.

The diet is high in fat and low in carbohydrate and is designed to produce ketone bodies as a result of the incomplete oxidation of fat.

In order to produce ketosis the usual ratio of fat to protein and carbohydrate (1:3) in the diet is gradually reversed. The time usually required to achieve a reversed ratio (3:1) is 4 days. If the ketogenic-antiketogenic ratio of the final diet does not produce ketosis, a further increase in the amount of fat and a decrease in the amount of carbohydrate may be necessary.

The physician may wish to prescribe vitamin and mineral supplements, since the diet may not be adequate according to the Recommended Daily Dietary Allowances of the National Research Council for children.

DIETARY REQUIREMENTS OF KETOGENIC DIET

The dietary requirements are calculated as follows:

Calories.   The calorie level of the diet may be modified according to the appetite, rate of growth, and body weight of the child. Suggested calories per kilogram of ideal body weight are given. Calories may be rounded to the nearest hundred, if desired.

Age, year	Calories per kilogram of ideal body weight
1 to 3	100 to 80
3 to 5	80 to 60
5 to 10	75 to 55
10 to 15	55 to 40

Ketogenic-Antiketogenic Ratio (K:AK).   Reversing the ratio of protein and carbohydrate to fat may be achieved in 4 days. The ketogenic-antiketogenic ratio may be altered as suggested in the following table. The physician may indicate a different progression rate and ketogenic-antiketogenic ratio if desired.

Day	K:AK
First	1.1:1
Second	1.6:1
Third	2.2:1
Fourth	2.8:1

Protein.   For a patient 3 years of age or less—1.5 gm per kilogram of ideal body weight. For a patient more than 3 years of age—1.0 gm per kilogram of ideal body weight.

Carbohydrate.   Determined by subtracting grams of protein from total value allowed for carbohydrate and protein. See Ketogenic Calculation Table (page 119) or note procedure described on page 115.

The carbohydrate level should not be reduced below 10 gm. For some patients it may be necessary to decrease carbohydrate at a slower rate if intolerance to fat is exhibited.

Fat.   Note procedure described on page 115 or see the Ketogenic Calculation Table (page 119).

CALCULATION OF KETOGENIC DIET

The 4-day dietary regimen of fat (F) and of protein and carbohydrate (P+C) may be calculated as follows:

First day

To calculate for a ketogenic-antiketogenic ratio of 1.1:1
1 Gm F   = 9 Cal × 1.1 = 9.9 Cal
1 Gm P+C = 4 Cal × 1.0 = 4.0 Cal
13.9 Cal per unit

Second day

To calculate for a ketogenic-antiketogenic ratio of 1.6:1
1 Gm F   = 9 Cal × 1.6 = 14.4 Cal
1 Gm P+C = 4 Cal × 1.0 = 4.0 Cal
18.4 Cal per unit

Third day

To calculate for a ketogenic-antiketogenic ratio of 2.2:1
1 Gm F   = 9 Cal × 2.2 = 19.8 Cal
1 Gm P+C = 4 Cal × 1.0 = 4.0 Cal
23.8 Cal per unit

Fourth day

To calculate for a ketogenic-antiketogenic ratio of 2.8:1
1 Gm F   = 9 Cal × 2.8 = 25.2 Cal
1 Gm P+C = 4 Cal × 1.0 = 4.0 Cal
29.2 Cal per unit

Protein, Fat, and Carbohydrate.   Protein, fat, and carbohydrate may be calculated as follows:

1. Determine total calorie requirement of the child
2. Divide total calories by calories per unit:

$$\frac{\text{Total calories}}{\text{Calories per unit}} = \text{Total units per day}$$

3. For grams of fat, multiply the number of units by K value in the ketogenic-antiketogenic ratio:

Number of units × K = grams of fat

4. For grams of protein and carbohydrate, multiply the number of units by AK value (1) in the ketogenic-antiketogenic ratio:

Number of units × AK(1) = grams of protein and carbohydrate

5. For grams of protein, determine the number of grams according to age and kilogram per body weight
6. For grams of carbohydrate, subtract the grams of protein in the diet from the total units per day

Total units per day − P = grams of carbohydrate

SAMPLE DETERMINATION OF KETOGENIC DIET

Patient: 8-year-old boy
Height: 4 feet 1 inch
Weight: 25 kg
Calories: 1,375 (25 kg × 55 Cal)

The values for the 4-day dietary regimen are calculated as follows:

First day

1,375 Cal ÷ 13.9 Cal = 99 units
F 99 × 1.1 = 109 gm
P+C = 99 × 1.0 = 99 gm
P (1 gm/kg) = 25 gm
C (99 − 25) = 74 gm

Second day

1,375 Cal ÷ 18.4 Cal = 75 units
F 75 × 1.6 = 120 gm
P+C = 75 × 1.0 = 75 gm
P (1 gm/kg) = 25 gm
C (75 − 25) = 50 gm

Third day

1,375 Cal ÷ 23.8 Cal = 58 units
F 58 × 2.2 = 128 gm
P + C = 58 × 1.0 = 58 gm
P (1 gm/kg) = 25 gm
C (58 − 25) = 33 gm

Fourth day

1,375 Cal ÷ 29.2 Cal = 47 units
F 47 × 2.8 = 132 gm
P + C = 47 × 1.0 = 47 gm
P (1 gm/kg) = 25 gm
C (47 − 25) = 22 gm

Calculated Values of Dietary Program for 8-Year-Old Child

Day	Protein gm	Fat gm	Carbohydrate gm	Calories	Ratio K:AK	Calories per unit*
First	25	109	74	1,377	1.1:1	13.9
Second	25	120	50	1,380	1.6:1	18.4
Third	25	128	33	1,384	2.2:1	23.8
Fourth	25	132	22	1,376	2.8:1	29.2

*Procedure for calculation, page 115.

PLANNING OF 4-DAY REGIMEN (See sample illustration for 8-year-old child, above)

APPROXIMATE COMPOSITION (10 to 15% Variation)

The approximate composition will vary slightly from the calculated values according to the foods included in the diet.

Day	Protein gm	Fat gm	Carbohydrate gm	Calories	Ratio, K:AK
First	28	110	75	1,406	1.1:1
Second	25	121	50	1,389	1.6:1
Third	24	130	31	1,390	2.2:1
Fourth	24	134	20	1,382	2.8:1

SUGGESTED SERVINGS OF FOOD EXCHANGES

Servings of food exchanges are suggested for each day. See Mayo Ketogenic Clinic Food Exchange List, pages 119 through 122, for amounts of specific foods allowed. Food in the diet must be weighed.

In planning the diet, the level of fat is increased while the carbohydrate content is decreased during the 4-day regimen. Protein should remain at approximately the same level.

SUGGESTED DAILY FOOD EXCHANGES (Mayo Clinic Ketogenic Food Exchange List, pages 119 through 122)

Day	Meat	Fat	Whipping cream	Bread*	Bread product	Vegetable	Fruit
First	2	10	3	3	...	2	4
Second	2	13	3	1½	...	2	3
Third	2	11	4	...	3	2	2
Fourth and following	2	12	4	...	2	2	1/2

*Bread exchange from the Mayo Clinic Food Exchange List, inside covers.

SUGGESTED MENU PATTERN

8-Year-Old Child (Mayo Clinic Ketogenic Food Exchange List, pages 119 through 122)

	First day	*Second day*	*Third day*	*Fourth day*
	Number of servings*			
Breakfast				
Fruit	1	1	1	1/2
Bread[†]	1	1	...	...
Bread product	...	...	1	1
Fat	2	3	3	3
Whipping cream	1	1	2	2
Noon Meal				
Meat	1	1	1	1
Bread[†]	1	...	...	...
Bread product	...	...	1	1
Vegetable	1	1	1	1
Fat	4	5	4	4
Whipping cream	1	1	1	1
Fruit	2	1	1/2	...
Evening Meal				
Meat	1	1	1	1
Bread[†]	1	1/2	...	...
Bread product	...	...	1	...
Vegetable	1	1	1	1
Fat	4	5	4	5
Whipping cream	1	1	1	1
Fruit	1	1	1/2	...

*All food is weighed.
[†]See Mayo Clinic Food Exchange List, inside covers.

CALCULATION OF KETOGENIC DIET

Instead of calculating each diet individually, the following Ketogenic Calculation Table may be used.

To use this table, proceed as follows:
1. Determine the calorie requirement
2. Check the ratio to be used
3. Grams of fat are given in column F
4. Grams of carbohydrate and protein are given in column C + P
5. Subtract number of grams of protein (page 115) required by the patient from the total number of C + P. The remaining number equals the number of grams of carbohydrate.

Ketogenic Calculation Table

Ketogenic-Antiketogenic Ratio

Calories	1.1:1 F* gm	1.1:1 C + P* gm	1.6:1 F* gm	1.6:1 C + P* gm	2.2:1 F* gm	2.2:1 C + P* gm	2.8:1 F* gm	2.8:1 C + P* gm
800	64	58	69	43	73	33	76	27
900	72	65	78	49	84	38	87	31
1,000	79	72	87	54	92	42	96	32
1,100	87	79	96	60	102	46	105	38
1,200	95	86	104	65	111	50	115	41
1,300	103	94	113	71	120	55	125	45
1,400	111	101	122	76	129	59	134	48
1,500	119	108	130	82	139	63	144	51
1,600	127	115	139	87	148	67	153	55
1,700	135	122	148	92	158	71	163	58
1,800	143	130	157	98	167	76	173	62
1,900	151	137	165	103	176	80	182	65
2,000	159	144	174	109	185	84	192	68
2,100	166	151	183	114	194	88	201	72
2,200	174	159	191	120	203	92	211	75

*F = fat; C + P = carbohydrate and protein.

EXCHANGE LIST FOR KETOGENIC DIET

The ketogenic diet is planned with the following Mayo Clinic Ketogenic Food Exchange List. The **Mayo Clinic Food Exchange List** (**inside covers**) **is not suitable** for planning ketogenic diets.

Mayo Clinic Ketogenic Food Exchange List (Average Values)

	Weight gm	Calories	Protein gm	Fat gm	Carbohydrate gm
Meat	30	73	7	5	...
Fat	5	36	...	4	...
Whipping Cream	60	187	2	19	2
Bread Products	2	7	...	...	1.6
Fruit	Varies	24	...	...	6
Vegetable					
A	100	16	1	...	3
B	50	16	1	...	3

MEAT EXCHANGE

One meat exchange is equivalent to
the weight listed and contains:

7 grams Protein
5 grams Fat
73 Calories

	Grams		Grams
Meat (medium fat)		**Fish**	
Beef, lamb, pork, or veal	30	Salmon or tuna, canned	30
Liver	30	Sardines	35
(add 1 fat exchange and		Shellfish	
omit 50 gm Veg A)		Clams	50
Sausage, pork	40	(add 1 fat exchange and	
(omit 2 fat exchanges)		omit 100 gm Veg A)	
Beef, dried	20	Lobster	40
(add 1 fat exchange)		(add 1 fat exchange)	
Bacon	25	Oysters	70
(omit 2 fat exchanges)		(add 1 fat exchange and omit	
Cold cuts	45	100 gm Veg A)	
Bologna, luncheon meat,		Scallops	50
minced ham, liverwurst		(add 1 fat exchange)	
(all meat, no cereal)		Shrimp	30
Salami	30	(add 1 fat exchange)	
(omit 1 fat exchange)			
Frankfurters or weiners (all meat,	50	**Cheese**	
no cereal)		American, brick, Cheddar, Roquefort	30
(omit 1 fat exchange)		Swiss, and processed cheese	
		(omit 1 fat exchange)	
Fowl		Cottage cheese, creamed	50
Chicken, duck, goose, or turkey	30	(add 1 fat exchange and omit 50	
		gm Veg A)	
Egg			
(one)			

FAT EXCHANGE

One fat exchange is equivalent to
the weight listed and contains:

4 grams Fat
36 Calories

	Grams		Grams
Avocado	30	Nuts	
(omit 50 gm Veg A)		Almonds, slivered	5
Butter or margarine	5	Pecans, shelled	5
Cooking fats	5	Walnuts, shelled	5
Mayonnaise	5	Oils, salad	5
		Olives, green or ripe	30

WHIPPING CREAM EXCHANGE

One whipping cream exchange is
60 grams and contains:

2 grams Protein
19 grams Fat
2 grams Carbohydrate
187 Calories

Whipping cream that is at least 32% fat should be used. Sixty (60) grams of whipping cream
may be exchanged for 65 grams of Vegetable A and 5 fat exchanges.

BREAD PRODUCTS

One bread product contains: 1.6 grams Carbohydrate
                                               7 Calories

Low calorie rice wafer—2 gm

FRUIT EXCHANGE (EP) *

One fruit exchange is equivalent to   6 grams Carbohydrate
the weight listed and contains: 24 Calories

	Grams			Grams
Apple		**Grapes**		
Fresh	40	Canned		40
Sauce	60	Fresh		40
Juice	60	Juice		
		Bottled		30
Apricots		Frozen		40
Canned	60			
Dried	10	**Lemon Juice**		75
Fresh	60			
Nectar	40	**Lime Juice**		65
Banana		**Mandarin Orange**		
Whole	30	Canned		100
Berries, fresh		**Mango**		
Blackberries	50	Fresh		35
Blueberries	40			
Boysenberries	60	**Melon**		
Cranberries	50	Cantaloupe		100
Gooseberries	60	Honeydew		100
Loganberries	50	Watermelon		100
Raspberries	50			
Strawberries	75	**Nectarine**		
		Fresh		40
Cherries				
Canned	60	**Orange**		
Fresh	40	Fresh, whole		50
		Juice		60
Dates		Sections, fresh or canned		50
Pitted	8			
		Papaya		
Figs		Fresh		60
Canned	60			
Dried	8	**Peach**		
Fresh	30	Canned		60
		Dried		10
Fruit Cocktail		Fresh		60
Canned	60	Nectar		60
Grapefruit		**Pear**		
Fresh	60	Canned		60
Juice	60	Dried		10
Sections, canned	75	Fresh		40
Nectar	40			

	Grams		Grams
Pineapple		**Prunes**	8
Canned	60	Juice	30
Fresh	40		
Juice	40	**Raisins**	8
Plums		**Rhubarb, raw**	160
Canned	60		
Fresh	40	**Tangerine**	
		Fresh, whole	50
		Juice	60
		Sections	50

*Edible portion only.

VEGETABLE EXCHANGE

One serving of Vegetable A or
Vegetable B contains:

1 gram Protein
3 grams Carbohydrate
16 Calories

Vegetable A 100 grams

Asparagus	Chard, Swiss	Peppers, green or red
Bean sprouts	Collards	Radishes
Beans, green or wax	Cress, garden	Sauerkraut
Beet greens	Cucumber	Spinach
Broccoli	Dill pickle	Squash, summer
Cabbage	Eggplant	Tomato juice
Cabbage, Chinese	Endive	Tomatoes
Cauliflower	Lettuce	Turnip greens
Celery	Mushrooms	Turnips
	Mustard greens	Watercress

Vegetable B 50 grams

Artichokes	Kale	Onions
Beets	Kohlrabi	Pumpkin
Brussels sprouts	Leeks	Rutabagas
Carrots	Okra	Squash, winter
Dandelion greens		

SODIUM-RESTRICTED DIETS

GENERAL INFORMATION

The milliequivalents of sodium in Sodium-Restricted Diets vary with each patient. The diet is based on the total number of calories necessary for the child to maintain a normal weight. The physician may order a diet with 1 mEq sodium per 100 calories or a diet with 4 mEq sodium per 100 calories. It is necessary for the physician to specify the child's weight in order to determine the calorie level of the diet.

CALCULATION OF SODIUM-RESTRICTED DIETS

A guide for the calculation of calorie levels of Sodium-Restricted Diets for hospitalized children follows. A hospitalized child usually does not require the number of calories recommended for a child who is healthy and active.

Kilograms of body weight	Calorie requirement
0 to 10	100 Cal per kilogram
10 to 20	1,000 Cal + 50 Cal for each kilogram over 10
20 or more	1,500 Cal + 20 Cal for each kilogram over 20

A *strict* or a *mild* sodium-restricted diet may be ordered using the following guide for calculation of sodium.

Approximate number of calories	Strict restriction, 1 mEq/100 calories	Mild restriction, 4 mEq/100 calories
1,000 or less	10 or less	40 or less
1,000 to 1,500	10 to 15*	40 to 60*
1,500 or more	15 to 25*	60 to 90*

*Hospital diets for children should not exceed the specified upper limits.

PLANNING OF SODIUM-RESTRICTED DIETS

Sodium-Restricted Diets should be planned to meet the Recommended Daily Dietary Allowance of the National Research Council for children. The protein level of the diet may vary according to the sodium restriction. When a high protein diet is ordered, substitution of dialyzed or low sodium milk or reduction of the amount of milk may be necessary in order to increase the protein content.

Parents of children who are to follow Sodium-Restricted Diets of 20 mEq or less at home are advised to check the sodium level of their local water supply. If the sodium level exceeds 1 mEq per quart, distilled water should be used. Chemically softened water should not be used on any sodium-restricted diet.

Sodium-Restricted Diet.   Sample Determination

Patient: 8-year-old child
　　　　Weight: Actual—25 kg

Calculation of calories: 1,500 calories + 20 Cal for each kilogram of weight over 20 kg

Diet: 1,600 calories

Strict Sodium Diet.   16 mEq (1 mEq/100 calories)

Mild Sodium Diet.   64 mEq (4 mEq/100 calories)

APPROXIMATE COMPOSITION (10 to 15% Variation)

Diet	Protein gm	Fat gm	Carbohydrate gm	Calories	Sodium mEq	Potassium mEq	Fluid ml
Strict Sodium (16 mEq)	55	70	190	1,610	17	70	1,200
Mild Sodium (64 mEq)	55	70	190	1,610	68	70	1,200

SUGGESTED DIET PATTERN

The Sodium-Restricted Diets for children are planned with the Mayo Clinic Food Exchange List. Servings of food exchanges for the sample illustration are suggested in the following table. Because an adequate caloric intake is important for each child, consideration should be given to food preferences.

SUGGESTED DAILY FOOD EXCHANGES (Mayo Clinic Food Exchange List, inside covers)

Diet	Meat	Fat	Milk	Bread	Vegetable	Fruit	Dessert
Strict Sodium (16 mEq)	3	5*	2	6	2	3*	1*
All foods processed or prepared without salt							
Mild Sodium (64 mEq)	3	5*	2	6*	2	3*	1*

Meat and vegetables unsalted; other foods processed or prepared with a moderate amount of salt.

*Amounts (unsalted) not restricted.

SUGGESTED MENU PATTERN (8-year-old child—1,600 calories)

	Strict Sodium Diet (16 mEq)	Mild Sodium Diet (64 mEq)
Breakfast		
Fruit	1 serving	1 serving
Cereal	1 serving	1 serving*
Bread	1 slice	1 slice*
Fat	1 teaspoon	1 teaspoon*
Milk	1/2 cup	1/2 cup
Sugar, jelly	1 tablespoon	1 tablespoon
Noon Meal		
Meat	1 ounce	2 ounces
Potato	1 serving	1 serving*
Vegetable	1 serving	1 serving
Bread	1 slice	1 slice*
Fat	2 teaspoons	2 teaspoons*
Fruit	1 serving	1 serving
Dessert	1 serving	1 serving
Milk	1 cup	1 cup
Evening Meal		
Meat	1 ounce	1 ounce
Potato	1 serving	1 serving*
Vegetable or salad	1 serving	1 serving
Bread	1 slice	1 slice*
Fat	2 teaspoons	2 teaspoons*
Fruit	1 serving	1 serving
Milk	1/2 cup	1/2 cup

*Foods processed or prepared with a moderate amount of salt.

AVERAGE SODIUM VALUES OF FOOD GROUPS

Average sodium values of food groups are listed in the following table for calculation of Sodium-Restricted Diets for children. See page 144 for table Sodium and Potassium Content of Foods in Mayo Clinic Food Exchange List if greater accuracy is desired.

Food	Amount	Sodium, mEq	
		Unsalted food	Salted food
Egg	1	3.0	5.0
Meat	1 ounce	1.0	3.0*
Fat	1 teaspoon	...	2.0
Milk	1 cup	...	5.0
Bread	1 serving	0.5	6.0
Potato or substitute	1/2 cup	0.5	10.0†
Vegetable	1/2 cup	0.5	10.0†

*Moderately salted during preparation; approximately 1/2 teaspoon per pound of meat.
†Moderately salted during preparation or processing; approximately 1/8 teaspoon per serving.

FOOD GROUPS

Allowed	Omitted
	Food preserved or prepared with salt except where allowed on specific diets (General Information, page 123)

Beverage

Allowed	Omitted
Coffee, tea, if permitted by the physician; soft drinks or carbonated beverages* (if less than 1 mEq of sodium per 8 ounces); cereal beverage	

Meat

Allowed	Omitted
Unsalted meat, fowl, liver, heart, egg, cheese, or peanut butter; fish, fresh clams, oysters, or shrimp (for child 6 years of age or less — fine bones removed)	Salted meat, fish, fowl, cheese, peanut butter; other organ meats; commercially frozen fish; other shellfish

Fat

Allowed	Omitted
Any unsalted except "Omitted" (for child 6 years of age or less — no nuts)	Salted butter, margarine; salad dressings; bacon; olives; salted nuts

Milk

Allowed	Omitted
Any except "Omitted"	Buttermilk, chocolate or malted milk, condensed milk

Bread

Allowed	Omitted
Salt-free bread, quick breads or rolls made with the following leavening agents: cream of tartar, potassium bicarbonate, sodium-free baking powder, yeast; unsalted crackers	Any made with salt, baking powder, or baking soda; commercially prepared mixes; self-rising flour
Unsalted cooked cereal; ready-to-eat cereal without salt	Instant, quick-cooking or ready-to-eat cereals with salt or sodium compound added*
Unsalted potato and potato substitutes	Commercially prepared mixes; potato chips; commercially frozen lima beans or peas; dried legumes; hominy; salted popcorn

Vegetable

Allowed	Omitted
Unsalted canned, cooked, fresh, or frozen except "Omitted"; no more than **one** serving daily of the following:	Any prepared with salt or sodium compounds

Artichokes	Collards
Beet greens	Dandelion greens
Beets	Kale
Carrots	Mustard
Celery	Spinach
Chard, Swiss	White turnips

Allowed	Omitted

Fruit

Any canned, dried, fresh, or frozen (for child 6 years of age or less—no pits or seeds)

Soup

Unsalted soup or broth; cream soup made with milk allowance

Any other

Dessert

Unsalted cake and cookies made with the following leavening agents: cream of tartar, potassium bicarbonate, sodium-free baking powder; unsalted pie; sodium-free gelatin*; pudding or frozen dairy dessert when used as part of milk allowance

Desserts made with baking powder, baking soda, or salt; commercial dessert mixes

Sweets

Sugar, honey; jam, jelly, marmalade without a sodium preservative*; plain sugar candy

Chocolate and cream candies

Miscellaneous

Pepper, spices and herbs except "Omitted"; flavoring extracts; bitter or sweet chocolate, cocoa powder; vinegar; unsalted white sauce; unsalted meat sauces

Salt or seasoned salts, mixed spices, dried celery products; bottled meat sauces, meat tenderizer, monosodium glutamate; pickles; milk chocolate, chocolate syrup, instant cocoa mix; gravy; regular baking powder, baking soda, salt substitutes unless approved by physician

*Consult list of ingredients on label or check with manufacturer.

APPENDIX

Recommended Daily Dietary Allowances,[a] Revised 1968.

Age[b] From–Up to	Weight		Height		Kilocalories	Protein	Fat-Soluble Vitamins			Water-Soluble Vitamins							Minerals				
							A activity	D	E activity	Ascorbic acid	Folacin[c]	Niacin	Ribo-flavin	Thi-amine	Vita-min B6	Vitamin B12	Cal-cium	Phos-phorus	Iodine	Iron	Magne-sium
years	kg	(lb)	cm	(in)	gm	gm	IU	IU	IU	mg	mg	mg equiv[d]	mg	mg	mg	mcg	gm	gm	µg	mg	mg
Infants																					
Birth–1/6	4	(9)	55	(22)	kg.×120[e]	kg.×2.2	1,500	400	5	35	0.05	5	0.4	0.2	0.2	1.0	0.4	0.2	25	6	40
1/6–1/2	7	(15)	63	(25)	kg.×110[e]	kg.×2.0	1,500	400	5	35	0.05	7	0.5	0.4	0.3	1.5	0.5	0.4	40	10	60
1/2–1	9	(20)	72	(28)	kg.×100[e]	kg.×1.8	1,500	400	5	35	0.1	8	0.6	0.5	0.4	2.0	0.6	0.5	45	15	70
Children																					
1–2	12	(26)	81	(32)	1,100	25	2,000	400	10	40	0.1	8	0.6	0.6	0.5	2.0	0.7	0.7	55	15	100
2–3	14	(31)	91	(36)	1,250	25	2,000	400	10	40	0.2	8	0.7	0.6	0.6	2.5	0.8	0.8	60	15	150
3–4	16	(35)	100	(39)	1,400	30	2,500	400	10	40	0.2	9	0.8	0.7	0.7	3	0.8	0.8	70	10	200
4–6	19	(42)	110	(43)	1,600	30	2,500	400	10	40	0.2	11	0.9	0.8	0.9	4	0.8	0.8	80	10	200
6–8	23	(51)	121	(48)	2,000	35	3,500	400	15	40	0.2	13	1.1	1.0	1.0	4	0.9	0.9	100	10	250
8–10	28	(62)	131	(52)	2,200	40	3,500	400	15	40	0.3	15	1.2	1.1	1.2	5	1.0	1.0	110	10	250
Males																					
10–12	35	(77)	140	(55)	2,500	45	4,500	400	20	40	0.4	17	1.3	1.3	1.4	5	1.2	1.2	125	10	300
12–14	43	(95)	151	(59)	2,700	50	5,000	400	20	45	0.4	18	1.4	1.4	1.6	5	1.4	1.4	135	18	350
14–18	59	(130)	170	(67)	3,000	60	5,000	400	25	55	0.4	20	1.5	1.5	1.8	5	1.4	1.4	150	18	400
18–22	67	(147)	175	(69)	2,800	60	5,000	400	30	60	0.4	18	1.6	1.4	2.0	5	0.8	0.8	140	10	400
22–35	70	(154)	175	(69)	2,800	65	5,000	—	30	60	0.4	18	1.7	1.4	2.0	5	0.8	0.8	140	10	350
35–55	70	(154)	173	(68)	2,600	65	5,000	—	30	60	0.4	17	1.7	1.3	2.0	5	0.8	0.8	125	10	350
55–75+	70	(154)	171	(67)	2,400	65	5,000	—	30	60	0.4	14	1.7	1.2	2.0	6	0.8	0.8	110	10	350
Females																					
10–12	35	(77)	142	(56)	2,250	50	4,500	400	20	40	0.4	15	1.3	1.1	1.4	5	1.2	1.2	110	18	300
12–14	44	(97)	154	(61)	2,300	50	5,000	400	20	45	0.4	15	1.4	1.2	1.6	5	1.3	1.3	115	18	350
14–16	52	(114)	157	(62)	2,400	55	5,000	400	25	50	0.4	16	1.4	1.2	1.8	5	1.3	1.3	120	18	350
16–18	54	(119)	160	(63)	2,300	55	5,000	400	25	50	0.4	15	1.5	1.2	2.0	5	1.3	1.3	115	18	350
18–22	58	(128)	163	(64)	2,000	55	5,000	400	25	55	0.4	13	1.5	1.0	2.0	5	0.8	0.8	100	18	350
22–35	58	(128)	163	(64)	2,000	55	5,000	—	25	55	0.4	13	1.5	1.0	2.0	5	0.8	0.8	100	18	350
35–55	58	(128)	160	(63)	1,850	55	5,000	—	25	55	0.4	13	1.5	1.0	2.0	5	0.8	0.8	90	18	300
55–75+	58	(128)	157	(62)	1,700	55	5,000	—	25	55	0.4	13	1.5	1.0	2.0	6	0.8	0.8	80	10	300
Pregnancy					+ 200	65	6,000	400	30	60	0.8	15	1.8	+0.1	2.5	8	+0.4	+0.4	125	18	450
Lactation					+1,000	75	8,000	400	30	60	0.5	20	2.0	+0.5	2.5	6	+0.5	+0.5	150	18	450

[a] The allowance levels are intended to cover individual variations among most normal persons as they live in the United States under usual environmental stresses. The recommended allowances can be attained with a variety of common foods providing other nutrients for which human requirements have been less well defined.

[b] Entries on lines for age range 22-35 years represent the reference man and woman at age 22. All other entries represent allowances for the midpoint of the specified age range.

[c] The folacin allowances refer to dietary sources as determined by *Lactobacillus casei* assay. Pure forms of folacin may be effective in doses less than 1/4 of the RDA.

[d] Niacin equivalents include dietary sources of the vitamin itself plus 1 mg equivalent for each 60 mg of dietary tryptophan.

[e] Assumes protein equivalent to human milk. For proteins not 100% utilized, factors should be increased proportionately.

FOOD COMPOSITION TABLE

PROCEDURE USED TO DEVISE TABLE

Therapeutic and standard hospital diets were nutritionally analyzed by using the following Food Composition Table. The nutritive values listed in the Food Composition Table represent average weighted nutritive values of foods served on the cycle menus of the associated hospitals of the Mayo Clinic and of foods consumed by the average adult.

The daily diet for the average adult was determined by evaluation of the pamphlet "Food Consumption and Dietary Levels of Households in the United States, 1965," published by the Department of Agriculture. The amounts and kinds of foods consumed were analyzed.

			Food Composition Table.		Nutrient Values		
Food	Wt	Amount	Calories	Protein	Fat	CHO	Ca
	gm			gm	gm	gm	mg
Meat							
Meat, fish, fowl	30	1 oz	73	7	5	...	15
Meat substitute†	30	1 oz	116	8	9	2	97
Egg	50	1	73	7	5	...	28
Fat							
Butter, margarine	5	1 tsp	36	...	4	...	1
Salad dressing	15	1 T	62	...	6	2	2
Gravy, white sauce	50	1/4 cup	39	1	3	2	15
Half and half	30	2 T	36	...	4	...	32
Milk							
Whole milk	240	1 cup	170	8	10	12	283
Milk drink	200	1 cup	204	8	8	25	270
Eggnog	200	1 cup	295	15	15	25	300
Bread							
Bread	25	1 slice	69	2	1	13	21
Cereal	20	2/3 cup	69	2	1	13	30
Potato or substitute	100	1/2 cup	69	2	1	13	7
Vegetable							
A	150	1/2-2/3 cup	...	...	...	...	56
B	75	1/2 cup	24	1	...	5	20
Fruit							
Citrus	100	1/2 cup	48	...	...	12	15
Other	Varies	1 serving	84†	1	...	20†	8
Soup							
Cream	200	1 cup	69	2	1	13	140
Dessert							
Regular	Varies	1 serving	212	3	8	32	55
Modified	Varies	1 serving	189	4	5	32	90
Low fat	Varies	1 serving	128	2	...	30	10
Sugar							
Sugar, jelly	15	1 T	56	...	...	14	...

*Value is for average amount of salt used in preparation of food; salt which may be added to food at the table is not calculated.

†Egg, cheese, cottage cheese, peanut butter.

†Average value for a serving of fruit, sweetened or unsweetened.

Agriculture Handbook No. 8 was the only source of reference for nutritive values (see Preface, page iii). A computer was used in the calculation procedure.

Nutrient values from the three different food patterns (menus of the two associated hospitals and the average outpatient's diet) were averaged together. The Food Composition Table illustrates average nutritive value of foods normally consumed every day. Nutrient values of frequently used modified foods are included also.

All standard and therapeutic diets were nutritionally analyzed with the nutritive values in the Food Composition Table. For food in which a range in the number of servings was given, the minimal amount was used for calculation purposes. The chart may be used for quick calculation of the nutritional adequacy of a diet. When more accurate figures are desired, reference sources listing specific foods should be consulted.

of Foods in Hospital and Outpatient Diets

Fe gm	Vit A IU	Thiamine mg	Riboflavin mg	Niacin mg equiv	Ascorbic acid mg	Sodium* mEq	Potassium mEq	Fluid ml
1.0	350	.06	.15	2.0	...	3	3	20
0.4	159	.02	.10	1.6	...	7	2	20
1.1	585	.04	.13	...	...	3	3	35
...	165	...	...	...	...	2	...	1
...	...	...	...	...	...	9	...	5
0.2	40	.01	.04	...	...	4	1	20
...	144	.01	.04	...	...	1	1	24
...	336	.07	.41	0.3	2	5	9	209
1.0	425	.10	.36	0.3	2	6	9	160
1.5	940	.14	.56	3.7	3	7	10	...
0.6	...	.06	.05	0.6	...	6	1	9
0.6	...	.08	.05	0.6	...	6	1	112
0.6	...	.09	.04	1.5	16	10	5	80
1.6	2120	.08	.12	0.8	30	16	8	140
0.8	3190	.08	.06	0.8	10	10	4	65
0.2	130	.07	.03	0.2	40	...	4	90
0.5	340	.02	.03	0.4	4	...	4	82
0.8	985	.10	.20	1.1	...	35	7	180
0.3	155	.03	.08	0.2	...	6	2	40
0.4	180	.03	.10	0.4	...	6	2	80
...	...	.02	.06	0.1	...	6	2	50
...	...	...	...	...	...	...	...	...

VITAMIN SUPPLEMENTS

The vitamin supplements that may be prescribed by physicians are pharmaceutical preparations, usually in capsule form. The composition of the vitamin supplements should approximate that of the hexavitamin capsule of the *National Formulary XII*.

The capsule contains:

Vitamin A	1.5 mg	(5,000 U.S.P. units)
Vitamin D	10 mcg	(400 U.S.P. units)
Ascorbic acid	75 mg	
Thiamine hydrochloride	2 mg	
Riboflavin	3 mg	
Nicotinamide	20 mg	

NUTRITIVE VALUES

ALCOHOLIC AND CARBONATED BEVERAGES[1]

Beverage	Average amount	Calories	Carbohydrate gm	Alcohol* gm
Alcoholic beverages				
Beer	8 oz	100	9	9
Brandy[2]	Brandy glass	75	...	11
Gin, rum, vodka, whiskey				
80 proof	1 jigger	70	...	10
90 proof	1 jigger	80	...	11
100 proof	1 jigger	90	...	13
Liqueurs (average)[2]	Cordial glass	65	6	7
Wines[2]				
Champagne	$3\frac{1}{2}$ oz	75	3	10
Muscatel	$3\frac{1}{2}$ oz	160	14	15
Sauterne	$3\frac{1}{2}$ oz	85	4	10
Table type wine	$3\frac{1}{2}$ oz	85	...	10
Vermouth, French	$3\frac{1}{2}$ oz	105	1	15
Vermouth, Italian	$3\frac{1}{2}$ oz	165	12	18
Carbonated beverages				
Carbonated waters				
(sweetened quinine soda)	1 cup	75	19	...
Cola type	1 cup	95	24	...
Ginger ale	1 cup	75	19	...
Root beer	1 cup	100	25	...
Soda, cream, or fruit flavored	1 cup	105	26	...

*Alcohol calculated as 7 calories per gram.

1. Watt, Bernice K., and Merrill, Annabel L.: Composition of Foods: Raw, Processed, Prepared. Handbook No. 8. Washington, D.C., U.S. Department of Agriculture, 1963, 189 pp.
2. Bowes, Anna de Planter, and Church, C. F.: Food Values of Portions Commonly Used. (Edited by C. F. Church and Helen N. Church.) Ed. 10. Philadelphia, J. B. Lippincott Company, 1966, 154 pp.

DESSERTS AND SNACK FOODS

Food	Approximate amount	Protein gm	Fat gm	Carbohydrate gm	Calories
Bread					
Coffee cake	$4\frac{1}{2}''$ diam	3	5	26	160
Sweet roll	1 average	5	4	30	175
Cake					
Chocolate, iced	1 ($2''\times3''\times2''$)	2	5	33	185
Pound cake	1 ($3''\times3''\times1/2''$)	3	9	27	200
White, iced	1 ($2''\times3''\times2''$)	2	5	30	175
Candy (approximately 1 oz)					
Bar candy, chocolate covered	1-oz	3	8	20	165
Butterscotch	6 pieces	...	3	24	125
Caramels	3 medium	1	3	22	120
Chocolate					
Creams	2 average	1	4	18	110
Fudge	1 1/4'' square	1	3	24	127
Mints	3 small	1	4	23	130
Hard candy	6 squares	...	...	30	120
Peanut brittle	$2\frac{1}{2}''\times2\frac{1}{2}''$	2	4	18	115
Cookies					
Assorted	1 (2'' diam)	1	4	14	95
Brownies	1 ($2''\times2''$)	2	10	15	160
Doughnuts					
Cake type, plain	1	2	6	16	125
Yeast leavened, plain	1	2	8	11	125
Pudding					
Chocolate	1/2 cup	3	5	26	160
Vanilla	1/2 cup	4	4	16	115
Custard	1/2 cup	3	4	23	140
Pie					
Cream	1/6 of 9'' pie	7	15	60	400
Custard-type	1/6 of 9'' pie	9	15	35	310
Chiffon	1/6 of 9'' pie	7	13	45	325
Fruit	1/6 of 9'' pie	4	15	60	390
Soup					
Bean	1 cup	6	2	26	145
Beef	1 cup	6	4	12	110
Cream	1 cup	7	12	18	210
Vegetable	1 cup	4	2	14	90

ACID-BASE REACTION OF FOODS

POTENTIALLY ACID OR ACID-ASH FOODS

Meat
Meat, fish, fowl, shellfish
Eggs
Cheese, all types
Peanut butter

Fat
Bacon
Nuts: Brazil, filberts, peanuts, walnuts

Bread
Breads, all types; crackers
Macaroni, spaghetti, noodles

Vegetable
Corn and lentils

Fruit
Cranberries, plums, prunes

Dessert
Cakes and cookies, plain

POTENTIALLY BASIC OR ALKALINE-ASH FOODS

Milk, Cream, and Buttermilk

Nuts
Almonds, chestnuts, coconut

Vegetable
All types (except corn and lentils)

Fruit
All types (except cranberries, prunes, plums)

NEUTRAL FOODS

Fats
Butter or margarine
Cooking fats and oils

Sweets
Candy, plain
Sugar and syrup

Starch
Arrowroot, corn, tapioca

FATTY ACID AND CHOLESTEROL CONTENT OF FOODS

Food	Approximate amount	Weight gm	Total fat gm	Saturated fat gm	Unsaturated fatty acids Oleic gm	Linoleic gm	Cholesterol mg
Meat Group							
Beef	1 oz	30	7.5	3.6	3.3	Trace	27
Veal	1 oz	30	3.6	1.8	1.5	Trace	27
Lamb	1 oz	30	6.3	3.6	2.4	Trace	27
Pork, ham	1 oz	30	7.8	3.0	3.3	Trace	27
Liver	1 oz	30	1.5	0.4	Trace	Trace	75
Beef, dried	2 slices	20	1.2	0.6	0.6	...	18
Pork sausage	2 links	40	17.6	6.4	7.6	1.6	45
Cold cuts	1 slice	45	9.7	2.4	2.7	0.6	30
Frankfurters	1	50	17.4	9.0	8.0	0.4	50
Fowl	1 oz	30	3.6	1.2	1.2	0.6	23
Eggs	1	50	6.0	2.0	2.5	0.5	253
Fish	1 oz	30	2.7	0.5	1.7	0.5	21
Salmon and tuna	1/4 cup	30	5.1	1.4	1.5	1.2	...
Shellfish	1 oz	30	1.9	0.6	1.0	0.3	45
Cheese	1 oz	30	9.0	5.1	3.0	...	45
Cottage cheese	1/4 cup	50	2.1	1.0	0.5	...	5
Peanut butter	2 T	30	15.0	2.7	7.5	4.2	...
Peanuts	25	25	12.0	2.5	5.0	3.2	...
Fat Group							
Avocado	1/8	30	5.1	0.9	2.4	0.6	...
Bacon	1 strip	5	2.6	0.9	1.0	0.3	5
Butter	1 tsp	5	4.0	2.3	1.2	...	12
Margarine	1 tsp	5	4.0	1.1	2.5	0.4	...
Special margarine	1 tsp	5	4.0	0.6	2.3	1.1	...
Coconut oil	1 tsp	5	5.0	4.4	0.5	0.1	...
Corn oil	1 tsp	5	5.0	0.5	1.8	2.7	...
Cottonseed oil	1 tsp	5	5.0	1.3	1.2	2.5	...
Olive oil	1 tsp	5	5.0	0.6	4.0	0.4	...
Peanut oil	1 tsp	5	5.0	0.9	1.6	1.5	...
Safflower oil	1 tsp	5	5.0	0.4	1.0	3.6	...
Sesame oil	1 tsp	5	5.0	0.9	1.0	2.1	...
Soybean oil	1 tsp	5	5.0	0.8	1.6	2.6	...
Vegetable fat	1 tsp	5	5.0	1.0	2.6	0.4	...
Half and half	2 T	30	3.6	1.8	1.8	...	12
Cream substitute, dried	1 T	2	0.5	0.3	0.2	...	...
Whipping cream	1 T	15	5.6	3.2	2.2	0.2	18
Cream cheese	1 T	15	5.3	3.0	2.2	0.1	18
Mayonnaise	1 tsp	5	4.0	0.7	1.3	2.0	8
French dressing	1 T	15	5.0	1.1	1.1	3.0	...
Nuts							
Almonds	5	6	3.5	0.3	2.5	0.7	...
Pecans	4	5	3.6	0.3	2.6	0.7	...
Walnuts	5	10	6.5	0.4	2.0	4.0	...
Olives	3	30	4.2	0.6	3.0	0.3	...

Food	Approximate amount	Weight *gm*	Total fat *gm*	Saturated fat *gm*	Unsaturated fatty acids		Choles-terol *mg*
					Oleic *gm*	Linoleic *gm*	
Milk Group							
Milk, whole	1 cup	240	8.5	4.9	3.6	...	27
2% milk	1 cup	240	4.9	2.4	2.5	...	15
Skim milk	1 cup	240	...	...	...	...	7
Cocoa (skim milk)	1 cup	240	1.9	0.7	1.2	...	...
Chocolate milk	1 cup	240	8.5	2.5	6.0	...	...
Bread Group							
Bread	1 slice	25	0.8	0.3	0.5	...	...
Biscuit	1	35	6.5	2.3	3.4	0.8	17
Muffin	1	35	3.5	0.7	2.4	0.4	16
Cornbread	1 (1 1/2″ cube)	35	4.0	1.4	2.1	0.4	16
Roll	1	28	1.3	0.3	0.7	0.3	...
Pancake	1 (4″ diam)	45	3.2	0.9	1.9	0.4	38
Waffle	1	35	3.4	1.0	2.1	0.4	28
Sweet roll	1	35	8.2	2.4	5.1	0.7	25
French toast	1 slice	65	8.1	3.9	3.4	0.8	130
Doughnut	1	30	6.0	1.3	4.4	0.3	27
Cereal, cooked	2/3 cup	140	1.4	...	1.4	0.3	...
Crackers (saltines)	6	20	2.4	0.6	1.4	...	...
Popcorn (unbuttered)	1 cup	15	0.7	0.1	0.2	0.4	...
Potatoes							
Potato chips	1–oz bag	30	12.0	3.0	4.0	6.0	...
French fried							
In corn oil	10	50	6.2	0.4	2.3	3.5	...
In hydroge-nated fat	10	50	6.2	1.6	4.0	0.6	...
Mashed potato	1/2 cup	100	4.3	2.0	2.3	...	...
Soup, cream	1/2 cup	100	4.2	1.0	2.2	1.0	9
Dessert							
Ice milk	1/2 cup	75	2.5	1.5	...	...	5
Ice cream	1/2 cup	75	9.0	5.0	3.9	...	43
Sherbet	1/3 cup	50	0.6	0.4	0.2	...	...
Low fat cookies	5	15	1.8	0.3	...	...	...
Cake	1 piece	50	14.0	2.0	...	0.5	45
Fruit pie	1/6 pie (9″)	160	15.0	4.0	9.5	1.4	11
Miscellaneous							
Gravy	1/4 cup	60	13.8	6.8	6.6	0.4	18
White sauce	1/4 cup	60	8.2	4.6	3.6	...	29
Coconut	1 oz	28	10.9	9.5	1.4	...	...
Chocolate sauce	1 oz	30	3.8	2.0	1.8	...	...

CALCULATION OF RATIO OF POLYUNSATURATED TO SATURATED FATS
IN CHOLESTEROL – CONTROLLED DIETS
SHORT METHOD

Food group	Approximate amount	Weight gm	Total fat gm	Saturated fat gm	Linoleic acid gm
Meat, fish, fowl, cooked	1 ounce	30	5	2.2	0.3
Eggs	2 wk	14	2	0.6	0.1
Bread	1 slice	25	1	0.3	...
Margarine					
Safflower oil	1 teaspoon	5	4	0.6	2.2
Corn oil	1 teaspoon	5	4	0.9	1.3
Vegetable oils					
Corn oil	1 teaspoon	5	5	0.3	2.5
Cottonseed oil	1 teaspoon	5	5	1.4	2.5
Safflower oil	1 teaspoon	5	5	0.3	3.5
Soybean oil	1 teaspoon	5	5	0.7	2.5
Salad dressing					
Mayonnaise	1 teaspoon	5	4	0.7	2.0
Other dressing	1 teaspoon	5	2	0.4	1.0

MEDIUM CHAIN TRIGLYCERIDES

Medium chain triglycerides (MCT) are a mixture of triglycerides synthesized from a distillate of coconut oil containing fatty acids with a chain length varying from 6 to 12 carbon atoms. Currently, and for present purposes, medium chain triglycerides are considered adjunctive nutritional therapy. Their physiology and clinical applications have been comprehensively covered in recent reviews.

The general areas in which medium chain triglycerides are considered clinically useful include certain malabsorptive disorders resulting from inadequate absorptive surface, disorders of intestinal lymphatic transport, bacterial overgrowth in the small intestine, and various inflammatory or infiltrative diseases of the small bowel. Medium chain triglycerides represent a concentrated source of calories, are more readily absorbed than dietary long chain triglycerides (LCT) under a variety of experimental and clinical conditions, and, at the same time, reduce fecal losses of water, electrolytes, and other nutrients. Medium chain triglycerides are not a substitute for proved specific therapy, but they are indicated in malabsorptive disorders for which specific therapy is unavailable or in which conventional therapy is only partially or temporarily effective.

Two principal forms of medium chain triglycerides are available commercially for therapeutic use: (1) The powdered formula, when prepared according to manufacturers' directions, provides 30 Cal per fluid ounce and 45 gm of fat per quart. (2) The medium chain triglyceride oil, which is liquid at room temperature, contains approximately 230 Cal in 30 ml (8.3 Cal per gram).

Fatty Acid Composition of Medium Chain Triglycerides[1]

	Fatty acid	MCT oil % of total fat	MCT powdered-formula diet % of total fat
$C_{6:0}$	Caproic	1	1
$C_{8:0}$	Caprylic; octanoic	75	71
$C_{10:0}$	Capric; decanoic	23	22
$C_{12:0}$	Lauric	1	1
$C_{14:0}$	Myristic	...	...
$C_{16:0}$	Palmitic	...	2
$C_{18:0}$	Stearic	Trace	...
$C_{18:1}$	Oleic	...	...
$C_{18:2}$	Linoleic	...	3

[1]Greenberger, N. J., and Skillman, T. G.: Medium-chain triglycerides: Physiologic considerations and clinical implications. New Eng. J. Med. 280:1045–1058 (May 8) 1969.

For additional information:

Holt, P. R.: Medium chain triglycerides: Useful adjunct in nutritional therapy. Gastroenterology 53:961–966 (Dec.) 1967.

Schizas, Alyette A., Cremen, Judith A., Larson, Elin, and O'Brien, Ruth: Medium-chain triglycerides—Use in food preparation. J. Amer. Dietet. Ass. 51:228–232 (Sept.) 1967.

Senior, J. R.: Medium Chain Triglycerides. Philadelphia, Division of Graduate Medicine, University of Pennsylvania, 1968, 300 pp.

FOODS HIGH IN CALCIUM

(More Than 25 Milligrams Calcium per Serving)

Food	Approximate amount	Weight *gm*	Calcium *mg*
Meat Group			
Egg	1	50	27
Fish			
Salmon (with bones)	1 oz	30	51
Sardines	1 oz	30	115
Clams	1 oz	30	29
Oysters	1 oz	30	31
Shrimp	1 oz	30	35
Cheese			
Cheddar	1 oz	30	218
Cheese foods	1 oz	30	160
Cheese spread	1 oz	30	158
Cottage cheese	1/4 cup	50	53
Fat			
Cream			
Half and half	2 T	30	32
Sour	2 T	30	31
Bread Group			
Bread			
Biscuit	2″ diameter	35	42
Muffin	2″ diameter	35	36
Cornbread	1 1/2 cube	35	36
Pancake	4″ diameter	45	45
Waffle	1/2 square	35	39
Beans, dry (canned or cooked)	1/2 cup	90	45
Lima beans	1/2 cup	100	42
Parsnips	2/3 cup	100	45
Milk			
Whole	1 cup	240	288
Evaporated whole milk	1/2 cup	120	302
Powdered whole milk	1/2 cup	30	252
Buttermilk	1 cup	240	296
Skim milk	1 cup	240	298
Powdered skim milk, dry	1/4 cup	30	367

FOODS HIGH IN CALCIUM

Food	Approximate amount	Weight *gm*	Calcium *mg*
Fruit			
Blackberries	3/4 cup	100	32
Orange	1 medium	100	41
Raspberries	3/4 cup	100	30
Rhubarb	1 cup	100	96
Tangerine	2 small	100	40
Vegetable A, cooked			
Beans, green or wax	1/2 cup	100	50
Beet greens	1/2 cup	100	99
Broccoli	1/2 cup	100	88
Cabbage	1/2 cup	100	49
Cabbage, Chinese	1/2 cup	100	43
Celery	1/2 cup	100	39
Chard	1/2 cup	100	73
Collards	1/2 cup	100	188
Cress	1/2 cup	100	81
Dandelion greens	1/2 cup	100	140
Mustard greens	1/2 cup	100	138
Sauerkraut	1/2 cup	100	36
Spinach	1/2 cup	100	93
Squash, summer	1/2 cup	100	25
Turnip greens	1/2 cup	100	184
Turnips	1/2 cup	100	35
Vegetable B, cooked			
Artichokes	1/2 cup	100	51
Brussels sprouts	1/2 cup	100	32
Carrots	1/2 cup	100	33
Kale	1/2 cup	100	187
Kohlrabi	1/2 cup	100	33
Leeks, raw	3–4	100	52
Okra	1/2 cup	100	92
Pumpkin	1/2 cup	100	25
Rutabagas	1/2 cup	100	59
Squash, winter	1/2 cup	100	28
Dessert			
Cake, white	1 piece	50	32
Custard, baked	1/3 cup	100	112
Ice cream	1/2 cup	75	110
Ice milk	1/2 cup	75	118
Pie, cream	1/6 of 9″ pie	160	120
Pudding	1/2 cup	100	117
Sherbet	1/3 cup	50	25

SODIUM AND POTASSIUM CONTENT OF FOODS
IN MAYO CLINIC FOOD EXCHANGE LIST

Food	Approximate amount	Weight gm	Sodium mEq	Potassium mEq
Meat				
Meat (cooked)				
Beef	1 ounce	30	0.8	2.8
Ham	1 ounce	30	14.3	2.6
Lamb	1 ounce	30	0.9	2.2
Pork	1 ounce	30	0.9	3.0
Veal	1 ounce	30	1.0	3.8
Liver	1 ounce	30	2.4	3.2
Sausage, pork	2 links	40	16.5	2.8
Beef, dried	2 slices	20	37.0	1.0
Cold cuts	1 slice	45	25.0	2.7
Frankfurters	1	50	24.0	3.0
Fowl				
Chicken	1 ounce	30	1.0	3.0
Goose	1 ounce	30	1.6	4.6
Duck	1 ounce	30	1.0	2.2
Turkey	1 ounce	30	1.2	2.8
Egg	1	50	2.7	1.8
Fish	1 ounce	30	1.0	2.5
Salmon				
Fresh	1/4 cup	30	0.6	2.3
Canned	1/4 cup	30	4.6	2.6
Tuna				
Fresh	1/4 cup	30	0.5	2.2
Canned	1/4 cup	30	10.4	2.3
Sardines	3 medium	35	12.5	4.5
Shellfish				
Clams	5 small	50	2.6	2.3
Lobster	1 small tail	40	3.7	1.8
Oysters	5 small	70	2.1	1.5
Scallops	1 large	50	5.7	6.0
Shrimp	5 small	30	1.8	1.7
Cheese				
Cheese, American or Cheddar type	1 slice	30	9.1	0.6
Cheese foods	1 slice	30	15.0	0.8
Cheese spreads	2 tablespoons	30	15.0	0.8
Cottage cheese	1/4 cup	50	5.0	1.1
Peanut butter	2 tablespoons	30	7.8	5.0
Peanuts, unsalted	25	25	…	4.5
Fat				
Avocado	1/8	30	…	4.6
Bacon	1 slice	5	2.2	0.6
Butter or margarine	1 teaspoon	5	2.2	…
Cooking fat	1 teaspoon	5	…	…

Food	Approximate amount	Weight gm	Sodium mEq	Potassium mEq
Cream				
Half and half	2 tablespoons	30	0.6	1.0
Sour	2 tablespoons	30	0.4	...
Whipped	1 tablespoon	15	0.3	1.0
Cream cheese	1 tablespoon	15	1.7	...
Mayonnaise	1 teaspoon	5	1.3	...
Nuts				
Almonds, slivered	5 (2 teaspoons)	6	...	0.8
Pecans	4 halves	5	...	0.8
Walnuts	5 halves	10	...	1.0
Oil, salad	1 teaspoon	5	...	...
Olives, green	3 medium	30	31.3	0.4
Bread				
Bread	1 slice	25	5.5	0.7
Biscuit	1 (2″ diameter)	35	9.6	0.7
Muffin	1 (2″ diameter)	35	7.3	1.2
Cornbread	1 (1 1/2″ cube)	35	11.3	1.7
Roll	1 (2″ diameter)	25	5.5	0.6
Bun	1	30	6.6	0.7
Pancake	1 (4″ diameter)	45	8.8	1.1
Waffle	1/2 square	35	8.5	1.0
Cereals				
Cooked	2/3 cup	140	8.7	2.0
Dry, flake	2/3 cup	20	8.7	0.6
Dry, puffed	1 1/2 cups	20	...	1.5
Shredded wheat	1 biscuit	20	...	2.2
Crackers				
Graham	3	20	5.8	2.0
Melba toast	4	20	5.5	0.7
Oyster	20	20	9.6	0.6
Ritz	6	20	9.5	0.5
Rye-Krisp	3	30	11.5	3.0
Saltines	6	20	9.6	0.6
Soda	3	20	9.6	0.6
Dessert				
Commercial gelatin	1/2 cup	100	2.2	...
Ice cream	1/2 cup	75	2.0	3.0
Sherbet	1/3 cup	50	...	...
Angel food cake	1 1/2″ × 1 1/2″	25	3.0	0.6
Sponge cake	1 1/2″ × 1 1/2″	25	1.8	0.6
Vanilla wafers	5	15	1.7	...
Flour products*				
Cornstarch	2 tablespoons	15	...	...
Macaroni	1/4 cup	50	...	0.8
Noodles	1/4 cup	50	...	0.6
Rice	1/4 cup	50	...	0.9
Spaghetti	1/4 cup	50	...	0.8
Tapioca	2 tablespoons	15	...	...
Vegetable*				
Beans, dried (cooked)	1/2 cup	90	...	10.0
Beans, lima	1/2 cup	90	...	9.5

Food	Approximate amount	Weight *gm*	Sodium *mEq*	Potassium *mEq*
Corn				
Canned[†]	1/3 cup	80	8.0	2.0
Fresh	1/2 ear	100	...	2.0
Frozen	1/3 cup	80	...	3.7
Hominy (dry)	1/4 cup	36	4.1	...
Parsnips	2/3 cup	100	0.3	9.7
Peas				
Canned[†]	1/2 cup	100	10.0	1.2
Dried	1/2 cup	90	1.5	6.8
Fresh	1/2 cup	100	...	2.5
Frozen	1/2 cup	100	2.5	1.7
Popcorn	1 cup	15	...	...
Potato				
Potato chips	1 oz	30	13.0	3.7
White, baked	1/2 cup	100	...	13.0
White, boiled	1/2 cup	100	...	7.3
Sweet, baked	1/4 cup	50	0.4	4.0
Milk				
Whole milk	1 cup	240	5.2	8.8
Evaporated whole milk	1/2 cup	120	6.0	9.2
Powdered whole milk	1/4 cup	30	5.2	10.0
Buttermilk	1 cup	240	13.6	8.5
Skim milk	1 cup	240	5.2	8.8
Powdered skim milk	1/4 cup	30	6.9	13.5
Vegetable A[*]				
Asparagus				
Cooked	1/2 cup	100	...	4.7
Canned[†]	1/2 cup	100	10.0	3.6
Frozen	1/2 cup	100	...	5.5
Bean sprouts	1/2 cup	100	...	4.0
Beans, green or wax				
Fresh or frozen	1/2 cup	100	...	4.0
Canned[†]	1/2 cup	100	10.0	2.5
Beet greens	1/2 cup	100	3.0	8.5
Broccoli	1/2 cup	100	...	7.0
Cabbage, cooked	1/2 cup	100	0.6	4.2
Raw	1 cup	100	0.9	6.0
Cauliflower, cooked	1 cup	100	0.4	5.2
Celery, raw	1 cup	100	5.4	9.0
Chard, Swiss	3/5 cup	100	3.7	8.0
Collards	1/2 cup	100	0.8	6.0
Cress, garden (cooked)	1/2 cup	100	0.5	7.2
Cucumber	1 medium	100	0.3	4.0
Eggplant	1/2 cup	100	...	3.8
Lettuce	Varies	100	0.4	4.5
Mushrooms, raw	4 large	100	0.7	10.6
Mustard greens	1/2 cup	100	0.8	5.5
Pepper, green or red				
Cooked	1/2 cup	100	...	5.5
Raw	1	100	0.5	4.0

Food	Approximate amount	Weight *gm*	Sodium *mEq*	Potassium *mEq*
Radishes	10	100	0.8	8.0
Sauerkraut	2/3 cup	100	32.0	3.5
Spinach	1/2 cup	100	2.2	8.5
Squash	1/2 cup	100	...	3.5
Tomatoes	1/2 cup	100	...	6.5
Tomato juice[†]	1/2 cup	100	9.0	5.8
Turnip greens	1/2 cup	100	0.7	3.8
Turnips	1/2 cup	100	1.5	4.8
Vegetable B*				
Artichokes	1 large bud	100	1.3	7.7
Beets	1/2 cup	100	1.8	5.0
Brussels sprouts	2/3 cup	100	...	7.6
Carrots, cooked	1/2 cup	100	1.4	5.7
Raw	1 large	100	2.0	8.8
Dandelion greens	1/2 cup	100	2.0	6.0
Kale, cooked	3/4 cup	100	2.0	5.6
Frozen	1/2 cup	100	1.0	5.0
Kohlrabi	2/3 cup	100	...	6.6
Leeks, raw	3–4	100	...	9.0
Okra	1/2 cup	100	...	4.4
Onions, cooked	1/2 cup	100	...	2.8
Pumpkin	1/2 cup	100	...	6.3
Rutabagas	1/2 cup	100	...	4.4
Squash, winter				
Baked	1/2 cup	100	...	12.0
Boiled	1/2 cup	100	...	6.5
Fruit				
Apple				
Fresh	1 small	80	...	2.3
Sauce	1/2 cup	120	...	2.5
Juice	1/2 cup	120	...	3.1
Apricots				
Canned	1/2 cup	120	...	6.0
Dried	4 halves	20	...	5.0
Fresh	3 small	120	...	8.0
Nectar	1/3 cup	80	...	3.0
Banana	1/2 small	60	...	4.8
Berries, fresh				
Blackberries	3/4 cup	100	...	3.0
Blueberries	1/2 cup	80	...	1.5
Boysenberries	1 cup	120	...	3.2
Gooseberries	3/4 cup	120	...	4.0
Loganberries	3/4 cup	100	...	4.4
Raspberries	3/4 cup	100	...	4.5
Strawberries	1 cup	150	...	6.3
Cherries				
Canned	1/2 cup	120	...	4.0
Fresh	15 small	80	...	2.7
Dates				
Pitted	2	15	...	2.5

Food	Approximate amount	Weight gm	Sodium mEq	Potassium mEq
Figs				
Canned	1/2 cup	120	...	4.6
Dried	1 small	15	...	2.5
Fresh	1 large	60	...	3.0
Fruit cocktail	1/2 cup	120	...	5.0
Grapes				
Canned	1/3 cup	80	...	2.2
Fresh	15	80	...	3.2
Juice				
Bottled	1/4 cup	60	...	2.8
Frozen	1/3 cup	80	...	2.4
Grapefruit				
Fresh	1/2 medium	120	...	3.6
Juice	1/2 cup	120	...	4.1
Sections	3/4 cup	150	...	5.1
Mandarin orange	3/4 cup	200	...	6.5
Mango	1/2 small	70	...	3.4
Melon				
Cantaloupe	1/2 small	200	...	13.0
Honeydew	1/4 medium	200	...	13.0
Watermelon	1/2 slice	200	...	5.0
Nectarine	1 medium	80	...	6.0
Orange				
Fresh	1 medium	100	...	5.1
Juice	1/2 cup	120		5.7
Sections	1/2 cup	100	...	5.1
Papaya	1/2 cup	120	...	7.0
Peach				
Canned	1/2 cup	120	...	4.0
Dried	2 halves	20	...	5.0
Fresh	1 medium	120	...	6.2
Nectar	1/2 cup	120	...	2.4
Pear				
Canned	1/2 cup	120	...	2.5
Dried	2 halves	20	...	3.0
Fresh	1 small	80	...	2.6
Nectar	1/3 cup	80	...	0.9
Pineapple				
Canned	1/2 cup	120	...	3.0
Fresh	1/2 cup	80	...	3.0
Juice	1/3 cup	80	...	3.0
Plums				
Canned	1/2 cup	120	...	4.5
Fresh	2 medium	80	...	4.1
Prunes	2 medium	15	...	2.6
Juice	1/4 cup	60	...	3.6
Raisins	1 tablespoon	15	...	2.9
Rhubarb	1/2 cup	100	...	6.5
Tangerines				
Fresh	2 small	100	...	3.2
Juice	1/2 cup	120	...	5.5
Sections	1/2 cup	100	...	3.2

*Value for products without added salt.
†Estimated average based on addition of salt, approximately 0.6% of the finished product.

CONVERSION TABLE

TO CONVERT MILLIGRAMS TO MILLIEQUIVALENTS

1. Divide milligrams by atomic weight

Example: 1,000 mg sodium $= \dfrac{1,000}{23} = 43.5$ mEq sodium

Mineral	Atomic weight
Sodium	23
Potassium	39

TO CONVERT SPECIFIC WEIGHT OF SODIUM TO SODIUM CHLORIDE

1. Multiply by 2.54

Example: 1,000 mg sodium $= 1,000 \times 2.54 = 2,540$ mg sodium chloride (2.5 gm)

TO CONVERT SPECIFIC WEIGHT OF SODIUM CHLORIDE TO SODIUM

1. Multiply by 0.393

Example: 2.5 gm sodium chloride $= 2.5 \times 0.393 = 1,000$ mg sodium

Milligrams	Sodium Values Milliequivalents	Grams of Sodium Chloride
500	21.8	1.3
1,000	43.5	2.5
1,500	75.3	3.8
2,000	87.0	5.0

MAYO CLINIC PHYSIOLOGIC VALUES

(Values Used by Mayo Clinic Physicians)

BLOOD VALUES

1. Energy (per 10 ml of blood)
   Carbohydrates
       Fasting sugar   65–90 mg
   Lipids (per 100 ml of plasma)
       Cholesterol, total   150–300 mg
       Cholesterol, esters   105–210 mg
       Phospholipids, total   180–320 mg
       Triglycerides $<$150–150 mg
2. Protein (per 100 ml of serum)
   Protein electrophoresis
       Albumin   3.3–4.3 gm
       Alpha–1–globulin   0.3–0.4 gm
       Alpha–2–globulin   0.5–0.8 gm
       Beta–globulin   0.6–1.1 gm
       Gamma–globulin   0.8–1.6 gm
   Urea (per 100 ml of blood)   Male 17–51 mg
        Female 13–45 mg
   Uric acid (per 100 ml of serum)   Male 4.3–8.0 mg
        Female 2.3–6.0 mg
   Phenylalanine (per 100 ml of plasma)   0.7–2.8 mg
3. Vitamins (per 100 ml of serum)
   Ascorbic acid   0.4–1.0 mg
   Carotene   48 μg
   Folic acid   5.9–16 mg
   Vitamin A   125–150 IU
4. Mineral elements (per 100 ml of serum)
   Calcium   8.9–10.1 mg
   Phosphorus   2.5– 4.5 mg
   Copper   75– 145 μg
   Protein-bound iodine   3.5– 7.5 μg
   Iron   75– 175 μg
   Magnesium   1.9– 2.6 mg
   Zinc   70– 140 μg
5. Electrolytes and water
   Carbon dioxide   25–29 mEq/liter of plasma
   Chloride   97–106 mEq/liter of plasma
   Potassium   4.0–5.0 mEq/liter of serum
   Sodium   135–145 mEq/liter of serum
   Osmolality   270–285 mOsm/liter of blood
6. Hematology
   Erythrocyte count   Male: 4,500,000–6,200,000/cu mm
        Female: 4,200,000–5,400,000/cu mm
   Hematocrit reading   Male: 42–54%
        Female: 38-46%
   Hemoglobin   Male: 14-17 gm/100 ml of blood
        Female: 12-15 gm/100 ml of blood
   Bleeding time   Duke: 1–5 min
        Ivy: 1–6 min

STOOL

Fat, quantitative	<7 gm/24 hr
Nitrogen	<2.5 gm/100 ml

URINE

Creatinine clearance	120–130 ml/min
Potassium	40–65 mEq/24 hr
Total protein excretion	<30 mg/24 hr
Sodium	130–200 mEq/24 hr
Urea clearance	40–60 ml/min
Uric acid	250–750 mg/24 hr

MISCELLANEOUS

Basal metabolism rate	-10 to $+10\%$
Schilling test	$>8\%$ excretion

HEIGHT-WEIGHT-AGE TABLES

PERCENTILES FOR WEIGHT AND HEIGHT

For Boys from Birth to 18 Years*

AGE	Percentiles						
	3	10	25	50	75	90	97
Birth							
Weight, pounds	5.8	6.3	6.9	7.5	8.3	9.1	10.1
Height, inches	18.2	18.9	19.4	19.9	20.5	21.0	21.5
3 mo.							
Weight, pounds	10.6	11.1	11.8	12.6	13.6	14.5	16.4
Height, inches	22.4	22.8	23.3	23.8	24.3	24.7	25.1
6 mo.							
Weight, pounds	14.0	14.8	15.6	16.7	18.0	19.2	20.8
Height, inches	24.8	25.2	25.7	26.1	26.7	27.3	27.7
9 mo.							
Weight, pounds	16.6	17.8	18.7	20.0	21.5	22.9	24.4
Height, inches	26.6	27.0	27.5	28.0	28.7	29.2	29.9
12 mo.							
Weight, pounds	18.5	19.6	20.9	22.2	23.8	25.4	27.3
Height, inches	28.1	28.5	29.0	29.6	30.3	30.7	31.6
15 mo.							
Weight, pounds	19.8	21.0	22.4	23.7	25.4	27.2	29.4
Height, inches	29.3	29.8	30.3	30.9	31.6	32.1	33.1
18 mo.							
Weight, pounds	21.1	22.3	23.8	25.2	26.9	29.0	31.5
Height, inches	30.5	31.0	31.6	32.2	32.9	33.5	34.7
2 yr.							
Weight, pounds	23.3	24.7	26.3	27.7	29.7	31.9	34.9
Height, inches	32.6	33.1	33.8	34.4	35.2	35.9	37.2
2 1/2 yr.							
Weight, pounds	25.2	26.6	28.4	30.0	32.2	34.5	37.0
Height, inches	34.2	34.8	35.5	36.3	37.0	37.9	39.2
3 yr.							
Weight, pounds	27.0	28.7	30.3	32.2	34.5	36.8	39.2
Height, inches	35.7	36.3	37.0	37.9	38.8	39.6	40.5
3 1/2 yr.							
Weight, pounds	28.5	30.4	32.3	34.3	36.7	39.1	41.5
Height, inches	37.1	37.8	38.4	39.3	40.3	41.1	41.9
4 yr.							
Weight, pounds	30.1	32.1	34.0	36.4	39.0	41.4	44.3
Height, inches	38.4	39.1	39.7	40.7	41.9	42.7	43.5
4 1/2 yr.							
Weight, pounds	31.6	33.8	35.7	38.4	41.4	43.9	47.4
Height, inches	39.6	40.3	40.9	42.0	43.3	44.2	45.0

*From Studies of Child Health and Development, Department of Maternal and Child Health, Harvard School of Public Health, and from Studies of Howard V. Meredith, Iowa Child Welfare Research Station, State University of Iowa, in the chapter of Stuart and Stevenson in Nelson: Pediatrics. 7th Ed. Philadelphia, W. B. Saunders Company, 1959.

PERCENTILES FOR WEIGHT AND HEIGHT

For Boys from Birth to 18 Years (Continued)

AGE	Percentiles						
	3	10	25	50	75	90	97
5 yr.							
Weight, pounds	33.6	35.5	37.5	40.5	44.1	46.7	50.4
Height, inches	40.2	40.8	41.7	42.8	44.2	45.2	46.1
5 1/2 yr.							
Weight, pounds		38.8	42.0	45.6	49.3	53.1	
Height, inches		42.6	43.8	45.0	46.3	47.3	
6 yr.							
Weight, pounds	38.5	40.9	44.4	48.3	52.1	56.4	61.1
Height, inches	42.7	43.8	44.9	46.3	47.6	48.6	49.7
6 1/2 yr.							
Weight, pounds		43.4	47.1	51.2	55.4	60.4	
Height, inches		44.9	46.1	47.6	48.9	50.0	
7 yr.							
Weight, pounds	43.0	45.8	49.7	54.1	58.7	64.4	69.9
Height, inches	44.9	46.0	47.4	48.9	50.2	51.4	52.5
7 1/2 yr.							
Weight, pounds		48.5	52.6	57.1	62.1	68.7	
Height, inches		47.2	48.6	50.0	51.5	52.7	
8 yr.							
Weight, pounds	48.0	51.2	55.5	60.1	65.5	73.0	79.4
Height, inches	47.1	48.5	49.8	51.2	52.8	54.0	55.2
8 1/2 yr.							
Weight, pounds		53.8	58.3	63.1	68.9	77.0	
Height, inches		49.5	50.8	52.3	53.9	55.1	
9 yr.							
Weight, pounds	52.5	56.3	61.1	66.0	72.3	81.0	89.8
Height, inches	48.9	50.5	51.8	53.3	55.0	56.1	57.2
9 1/2 yr.							
Weight, pounds		58.7	63.7	69.0	76.0	85.5	
Height, inches		51.4	52.7	54.3	55.9	57.1	
10 yr.							
Weight, pounds	56.8	61.1	66.3	71.9	79.6	89.9	100.0
Height, inches	50.7	52.3	53.7	55.2	56.8	58.1	59.2
10 1/2 yr.							
Weight, pounds		63.7	69.0	74.8	83.4	94.6	
Height, inches		53.2	54.5	56.0	57.8	58.9	
11 yr.							
Weight, pounds	61.8	66.3	71.6	77.6	87.2	99.3	111.7
Height, inches	52.5	54.0	55.3	56.8	58.7	59.8	60.8
11 1/2 yr.							
Weight, pounds		69.2	74.6	81.0	91.6	104.5	
Height, inches		55.0	56.3	57.8	59.6	60.9	
12 yr.							
Weight, pounds	67.2	72.0	77.5	84.4	96.0	109.6	124.2
Height, inches	54.4	56.1	57.2	58.9	60.4	62.2	63.7

PERCENTILES FOR WEIGHT AND HEIGHT

For Boys from Birth to 18 Years (Continued)

AGE	Percentiles						
	3	10	25	50	75	90	97
12 1/2 yr.							
Weight, pounds		74.6	80.6	88.7	102.0	116.4	
Height, inches		56.9	58.1	60.0	61.9	63.6	
13 yr.							
Weight, pounds	72.0	77.1	83.7	93.0	107.9	123.2	138.0
Height, inches	56.0	57.7	58.9	61.0	63.3	65.1	66.7
13 1/2 yr.							
Weight, pounds		82.2	89.6	100.3	115.5	130.1	
Height, inches		58.8	60.3	62.6	64.8	66.5	
14 yr.							
Weight, pounds	79.8	87.2	95.5	107.6	123.1	136.9	150.6
Height, inches	57.6	59.9	61.6	64.0	66.3	67.9	69.7
14 1/2 yr.							
Weight, pounds		93.3	101.9	113.9	129.1	142.4	
Height, inches		61.0	62.7	65.1	67.2	68.7	
15 yr.							
Weight, pounds	91.3	99.4	108.2	120.1	135.0	147.8	161.6
Height, inches	59.7	62.1	63.9	66.1	68.1	69.6	71.6
15 1/2 yr.							
Weight, pounds		105.2	113.5	124.9	139.7	152.6	
Height, inches		63.1	64.8	66.8	68.8	70.2	
16 yr.							
Weight, pounds	103.4	111.0	118.7	129.7	144.4	157.3	170.5
Height, inches	61.6	64.1	65.8	67.8	69.5	70.7	73.1
16 1/2 yr.							
Weight, pounds		114.3	121.6	133.0	147.9	161.0	
Height, inches		64.6	66.3	68.0	69.8	71.1	
17 yr.							
Weight, pounds	110.5	117.5	124.5	136.2	151.4	164.6	175.6
Height, inches	62.6	65.2	66.8	68.4	70.1	71.5	73.5
17 1/2 yr.							
Weight, pounds		118.8	125.8	137.6	153.6	166.8	
Height, inches		65.3	67.0	68.5	70.3	71.6	
18 yr.							
Weight, pounds	113.0	120.0	127.1	139.0	155.7	169.0	179.0
Height, inches	62.8	65.5	67.0	68.7	70.4	71.8	73.9

PERCENTILES FOR WEIGHT AND HEIGHT

For Girls from Birth to 18 Years*

AGE	Percentiles						
	3	10	25	50	75	90	97
Birth							
Weight, pounds	5.8	6.2	6.9	7.4	8.1	8.6	9.4
Height, inches	18.5	18.8	19.3	19.8	20.1	20.4	21.1
3 mo.							
Weight, pounds	9.8	10.7	11.4	12.4	13.2	14.0	14.9
Height, inches	22.0	22.4	22.8	23.4	23.9	24.3	24.8
6 mo.							
Weight, pounds	12.7	14.1	15.0	16.0	17.5	18.6	20.0
Height, inches	24.0	24.6	25.1	25.7	26.2	26.7	27.1
9 mo.							
Weight, pounds	15.1	16.6	17.8	19.2	20.8	22.4	24.2
Height, inches	25.7	26.4	26.9	27.6	28.2	28.7	29.2
12 mo.							
Weight, pounds	16.8	18.4	19.8	21.5	23.0	24.8	27.1
Height, inches	27.1	27.8	28.5	29.2	29.9	30.3	31.0
15 mo.							
Weight, pounds	18.1	19.8	21.3	23.0	24.6	26.6	29.0
Height, inches	28.3	29.0	29.8	30.5	31.3	31.8	32.6
18 mo.							
Weight, pounds	19.4	21.2	22.7	24.5	26.2	28.3	30.9
Height, inches	29.5	30.2	31.1	31.8	32.6	33.3	34.1
2 yr.							
Weight, pounds	21.6	23.5	25.3	27.1	29.2	31.7	34.4
Height, inches	31.5	32.3	33.3	34.1	35.0	35.8	36.7
2 1/2 yr.							
Weight, pounds	23.6	25.5	27.4	29.6	31.9	34.6	38.2
Height, inches	33.3	34.0	35.2	36.0	36.9	37.9	38.9
3 yr.							
Weight, pounds	25.6	27.6	29.6	31.8	34.6	37.4	41.8
Height, inches	34.8	35.6	36.8	37.7	38.6	39.8	40.7
3 1/2 yr.							
Weight, pounds	27.5	29.5	31.5	33.9	37.0	40.4	45.3
Height, inches	36.2	37.1	38.1	39.2	40.2	41.5	42.5
4 yr.							
Weight, pounds	29.2	31.2	33.5	36.2	39.6	43.5	48.2
Height, inches	37.5	38.4	39.5	40.6	41.6	43.1	44.2
4 1/2 yr.							
Weight, pounds	30.7	32.9	35.3	38.5	42.1	46.7	50.9
Height, inches	38.6	39.7	40.8	42.0	43.0	44.7	45.7
5 yr.							
Weight, pounds	32.1	34.8	37.4	40.5	44.8	49.2	52.8
Height, inches	39.4	40.5	41.6	42.9	44.0	45.4	46.8

*From Studies of Child Health and Development, Department of Maternal and Child Health, Harvard School of Public Health, and from Studies of Howard V. Meredith, Iowa Child Welfare Research Station, State University of Iowa, in the chapter of Stuart and Stevenson in Nelson: Pediatrics. 7th Ed. Philadelphia, W. B. Saunders Company, 1959.

PERCENTILES FOR WEIGHT AND HEIGHT

For Girls from Birth to 18 Years (Continued)

AGE	Percentiles						
	3	10	25	50	75	90	97
5 1/2 yr.							
Weight, pounds		38.0	40.8	44.0	47.2	51.2	
Height, inches		42.4	43.4	44.4	45.7	46.8	
6 yr.							
Weight, pounds	37.2	39.6	42.9	46.5	50.2	54.2	58.7
Height, inches	42.5	43.5	44.6	45.6	47.0	48.1	49.4
6 1/2 yr.							
Weight, pounds		42.2	45.5	49.4	53.3	57.7	
Height, inches		44.8	45.7	46.9	48.3	49.4	
7 yr.							
Weight, pounds	41.3	44.5	48.1	52.2	56.3	61.2	67.3
Height, inches	44.9	46.0	46.9	48.1	49.6	50.7	51.9
7 1/2 yr.							
Weight, pounds		46.6	50.6	55.2	59.8	65.6	
Height, inches		47.0	48.0	49.3	50.7	51.9	
8 yr.							
Weight, pounds	45.3	48.6	53.1	58.1	63.3	69.9	78.9
Height, inches	46.9	48.1	49.1	50.4	51.8	53.0	54.1
8 1/2 yr.							
Weight, pounds		50.6	55.5	61.0	66.9	74.5	
Height, inches		49.0	50.1	51.4	52.9	54.1	
9 yr.							
Weight, pounds	49.1	52.6	57.9	63.8	70.5	79.1	89.9
Height, inches	48.7	50.0	51.1	52.3	54.0	55.3	56.5
9 1/2 yr.							
Weight, pounds		54.9	60.4	67.1	74.8	84.4	
Height, inches		50.9	52.0	53.5	55.1	56.4	
10 yr.							
Weight, pounds	53.2	57.1	62.8	70.3	79.1	89.7	101.9
Height, inches	50.3	51.8	53.0	54.6	56.1	57.5	58.8
10 1/2 yr.							
Weight, pounds		59.9	66.4	74.6	84.1	95.1	
Height, inches		52.9	54.1	55.8	57.4	58.9	
11 yr.							
Weight, pounds	57.9	62.6	69.9	78.8	89.1	100.4	112.9
Height, inches	52.1	53.9	55.2	57.0	58.7	60.4	62.0
11 1/2 yr.							
Weight, pounds		66.1	74.0	83.2	94.0	106.0	
Height, inches		55.0	56.3	58.3	60.2	61.8	
12 yr.							
Weight, pounds	63.6	69.5	78.0	87.6	98.8	111.5	127.7
Height, inches	54.3	56.1	57.4	59.8	61.6	63.2	64.8
12 1/2 yr.							
Weight, pounds		74.7	83.7	93.4	104.9	118.0	
Height, inches		57.4	58.8	60.7	62.6	64.0	

PERCENTILES FOR WEIGHT AND HEIGHT

For Girls from Birth to 18 Years (Continued)

AGE	Percentiles						
	3	10	25	50	75	90	97
13 yr.							
Weight, pounds	72.2	79.9	89.4	99.1	111.0	124.5	142.3
Height, inches	56.6	58.7	60.1	61.8	63.6	64.9	66.3
13 1/2 yr.							
Weight, pounds		85.5	94.6	103.7	115.4	128.9	
Height, inches		59.5	60.8	62.4	64.0	65.3	
14 yr.							
Weight, pounds	83.1	91.0	99.8	108.4	119.7	133.3	150.8
Height, inches	58.3	60.2	61.5	62.8	64.4	65.7	67.2
14 1/2 yr.							
Weight, pounds		94.2	102.5	111.0	121.8	135.7	
Height, inches		60.7	61.8	63.1	64.7	66.0	
15 yr.							
Weight, pounds	89.0	97.4	105.1	113.5	123.9	138.1	155.2
Height, inches	59.1	61.1	62.1	63.4	64.9	66.2	67.6
15 1/2 yr.							
Weight, pounds		99.2	106.8	115.3	125.6	139.6	
Height, inches		61.3	62.3	63.7	65.1	66.4	
16 yr.							
Weight, pounds	91.8	100.9	108.4	117.0	127.2	141.1	157.7
Height, inches	59.4	61.5	62.4	63.9	65.2	66.5	67.7
16 1/2 yr.							
Weight, pounds		101.9	109.4	118.1	128.4	142.2	
Height, inches		61.5	62.5	63.9	65.3	66.6	
17 yr.							
Weight, pounds	93.9	102.8	110.4	119.1	129.6	143.3	159.5
Height, inches	59.4	61.5	62.6	64.0	65.4	66.7	67.8
17 1/2 yr.							
Weight, pounds		103.2	110.8	119.5	130.2	143.9	
Height, inches		61.5	62.6	64.0	65.4	66.7	
18 yr.							
Weight, pounds	94.5	103.5	111.2	119.9	130.8	144.5	160.7
Height, inches	59.4	61.5	62.6	64.0	65.4	66.7	67.8

GRADED AVERAGE WEIGHT

For Men of Ages 19 to 24 Years*

Height Without Shoes		Age, yr. at Last Birthday					
Feet	Inches	19	20	21	22	23	24
5	0	115	117	118	119	120	121
5	1	117	119	120	121	122	123
5	2	120	122	123	124	125	126
5	3	123	125	126	127	128	129
5	4	126	128	130	131	132	133
5	5	130	132	134	135	136	137
5	6	134	136	138	139	140	141
5	7	138	140	141	142	143	144
5	8	142	144	145	146	147	148
5	9	146	148	149	150	151	152
5	10	150	152	153	154	155	156
5	11	155	156	157	158	159	160
6	0	160	161	162	163	164	165
6	1	165	166	167	168	169	171
6	2	170	171	172	173	175	177
6	3	175	176	177	178	180	182
6	4	180	181	182	183	185	187
6	5	185	186	187	188	190	192

For Women of Ages 19 to 24 Years*

Height Without Shoes		Age, yr. at Last Birthday					
Feet	Inches	19	20	21	22	23	24
4	8	105	106	107	107	108	109
4	9	107	108	109	109	110	111
4	10	109	110	111	111	112	113
4	11	111	112	113	113	114	115
5	0	113	114	115	115	116	117
5	1	115	116	117	117	118	119
5	2	118	119	120	120	121	121
5	3	121	122	123	123	124	124
5	4	124	125	126	126	127	127
5	5	127	128	129	129	130	130
5	6	131	132	133	133	134	134
5	7	135	136	137	137	138	138
5	8	139	140	141	141	142	142
5	9	142	143	144	145	146	146
5	10	146	147	148	149	150	150
5	11	151	151	152	153	153	154
6	0	155	156	156	157	157	158

*Reprinted from Medico-Actuarial Mortality Investigation, Vol. 1, New York, 1912.

IDEAL WEIGHTS

For Men of Ages 25 Years or More*

Height in Shoes		Small Frame	Medium Frame	Large Frame
Feet	Inches			
5	2	112–120	118–129	126–141
5	3	115–123	121–133	129–144
5	4	118–126	124–136	132–148
5	5	121–129	127–139	135–152
5	6	124–133	130–143	138–156
5	7	128–137	134–147	142–161
5	8	132–141	138–152	147–166
5	9	136–145	142–156	151–170
5	10	140–150	146–160	155–174
5	11	144–154	150–165	159–179
6	0	148–158	154–170	164–184
6	1	152–162	158–175	168–189
6	2	156–167	162–180	173–194
6	3	160–171	167–185	178–199
6	4	164–175	172–190	182–204

For Women of Ages 25 Years or More*

Height in Shoes		Small Frame	Medium Frame	Large Frame
Feet	Inches			
4	10	92– 98	96–107	104–119
4	11	94–101	98–110	106–122
5	0	96–104	101–113	109–125
5	1	99–107	104–116	112–128
5	2	102–110	107–119	115–131
5	3	105–113	110–122	118–134
5	4	108–116	113–126	121–138
5	5	111–119	116–130	125–142
5	6	114–123	120–135	129–146
5	7	118–127	124–139	133–150
5	8	122–131	128–143	137–154
5	9	126–135	132–147	141–158
5	10	130–140	136–151	145–163
5	11	134–144	140–155	149–168
6	0	138–148	144–159	153–173

*Reprinted from Metropolitan Life Insurance Company, Stat. Bull. 40:1-12 (Nov. Dec.) 1959.

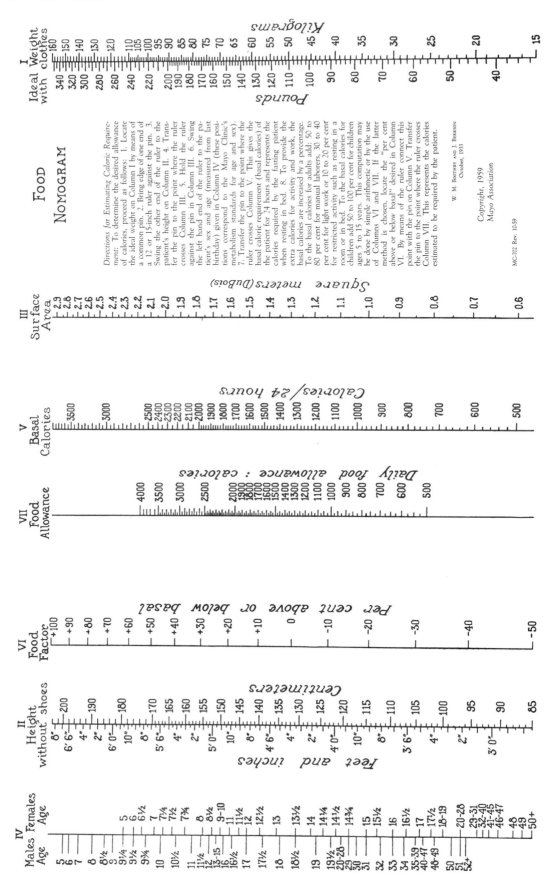

FOOD NOMOGRAM

Directions for Estimating Caloric Requirement: To determine the desired allowance of calories, proceed as follows: 1. Locate the ideal weight on Column I by means of a common pin. 2. Bring edge of one end of a 12 or 15-inch ruler against the pin. 3. Swing the other end of the ruler to the patient's height on Column II. 4. Transfer the pin to the point where the ruler crosses Column III. 5. Hold the ruler against the pin in Column III. 6. Swing the left hand end of the ruler to the patient's sex and age (measured from last birthday) given in Column IV (these positions correspond to the Mayo Clinic's metabolism standards for age and sex). 7. Transfer the pin to the point where the ruler crosses Column V. This gives the basal caloric requirement (basal calories) of the patient for 24 hours and represents the calories required by the fasting patient when resting in bed. 8. To provide the extra calories for activity and work, the basal calories are increased by a percentage. To the basal calories for adults add: 50 to 80 per cent for manual laborers; 30 to 40 per cent for light work or 10 to 20 per cent for restricted activity such as resting in a room or in bed. To the basal calories for children add 50 to 100 per cent for children ages 5 to 15 years. This computation may be done by simple arithmetic or by the use of Columns VI and VII. If the latter method is chosen, locate the "per cent above or below basal" desired in Column VI. By means of the ruler connect this point with the pin on Column V. Transfer the pin to the point where the ruler crosses Column VII. This represents the calories estimated to be required by the patient.

W. M. BOOTHBY AND J. BERKSON
October, 1933

Copyright, 1959
Mayo Association

MC-702 Rev. 10-59

I Ideal Weight with clothes — *Kilograms* / *Pounds*

III Surface Area — *Square meters (DuBois)*

V Basal Calories — *Calories/24 hours*

VII Food Allowance — *Daily food allowance : calories*

VI Food Factor — *Per cent above or below basal*

II Height without shoes — *Centimeters* / *Feet and inches*

IV Males Age / Females Age

BASAL CALORIC REQUIREMENTS OF CHILDREN

For a child less than 5 years of age, the basal caloric requirement for 24 hours is computed by multiplying the standard weight for the measured height by the basal requirement for calories per pound per 24 hours for the appropriate age (see the table which follows). The height is that of the child measured without shoes; the weight to be used is that in the "Woodbury Height-Weight-Age Table" which corresponds to the measured height and age of the child; the age to be used is that of the child to the nearest half year or full year.

Basal Requirement for Calories per Pound per 24 Hours

Age	Calories	
	Boys	Girls
6 months	25.0	25.0
1 year	25.5	25.5
2 years	25.0	24.5
3 years	23.5	23.5
4 years	23.0	22.0

INDEX